NATURE'S BEST REMEDIES

Earth Clinic Presents...

NATURE'S BEST REMEDIES

Edited by Daniel P. Kray

An Earth Clinic Publication

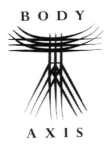

BODY

AXIS

Body Axis, LLC.
Atlanta

DISCLAIMER
The preparation and publication of this book has been undertaken with great care.
However, the book is offered for informational purposes only and cannot be taken
as a substitute for professional medical prevention, diagnosis, or treatment. Please
consult with your physician, pharmacist, or health care provider before taking any
home remedies or supplements or following any treatment suggested by anyone
within this book. Only your health care provider, personal physician, or pharmacist
can provide you with advice on what is safe and effective for your unique needs or
diagnose your particular medical history.

Visit us online at:
www.bodyaxis.com
www.earthclinic.com

Printed in the United States of America

FIRST PRINTING: 2011

ISBN-978-0-9828963-4-1

Table of Contents

C

D

E

F

G

H

N

O

P

Q-R

S

T

U

V

W

X-Z

INTRODUCTION

We're bringing you the very best that Earth Clinic has to offer in super-concentrated form—like a multivitamin of natural remedy knowledge! That's what this book is all about. More than a decade's worth of planet-spanning information on natural remedies has been collected on the pages of EarthClinic.com. It's the internet's most trusted resource for options in natural healing, it's wonderful, and it's colossal—sometimes overwhelmingly so.

Many of the natural remedies on Earth Clinic were passed down through generations. Others were discovered just yesterday to genuine fanfare on the website. Whatever the source of the knowledge, real people in the Earth Clinic Community have changed their lives with simple remedies from their own kitchens, their own gardens, and with other natural healing agents you can easily find not far from home. We at Earth Clinic are very proud to have built the sort of clinic where no one is turned away, where everyone returns home with more information and hopefully much improved in health.

Usually, they soon come back for more! Like we said, there is an enormous library of health secrets on the website, for those who are sick and in need just as well as for the hale and hearty who want to find the path to optimal health.

Sometimes though, all we want is the quick and easy answer. That can be especially true when we're sick or injured, or even more especially when those we love are the sick and injured. For that reason, the editors at Earth Clinic have distilled the vast Earth Clinic treasury of knowledge down to its best and essential answers to your home health needs in this book.

What is Earth Clinic?

In case you've never been to the Earth Clinic website, let me quickly explain what you will find here in this book. EarthClinic.com, an alternative health and healing site, was launched on the web in 1999. It has grown into a top-ranked health portal because people took an interest in the idea of simple, effective, tried-and-true remedies and in the possibility of freely sharing them with each other.

Earth Clinic has since become a global community of shared knowledge on safe, inexpensive, natural cures and home remedies from around the world. Each remedy has been contributed, tried, and reported on by regular people just like you. You and no one else! We do not accept direct advertising or promote any company's products. All we do is provide a venue for people to talk about their own family's experience with natural remedies used around the world. That's how you know you can trust us.

How We Chose Our Remedies

Reader contributions, with the input of a few alternative health expert volunteers, make up almost all of the material on the Earth Clinic website. Our in-house experts review and then allocate those contributions throughout the site to make up its content—hundreds of ailments matched by thousands of natural remedies.

In pulling this text together, we scanned all of the contributor posts for each condition, looking for those that had solid backing—many positive reports from readers who found a cure or relief in the remedy, and very few reports of side effects or incomplete cures (while remembering that no cure is going to work the same way for everyone).

Likewise, many conditions listed on the site were not included in the text you find here, simply because the jury is still out on finding a great natural remedy for that condition. You very well may find a remedy that works fabulously for you if you go and visit the site, but we wanted to present you with only the cream of the crop.

Only the absolute best remedies made the list to follow here. Still, that's not to say they're foolproof. Each person's health needs are different, even when suffering a common condition. But so many have found near-miraculous relief using these remedies that we are eager to share them as broadly and conveniently as possible.

A Word of Explanation

The remedies presented here are boiled down to the utmost simplicity—quick and handy answers to your pressing health needs. However, the treasury of first-person accounts on EarthClinic.com is hard to replace. Our brevity here is quick and efficient, but it necessarily neglects certain complexities presented in more detail online.

If you begin to find relief from a remedy presented in this book, or if you are having trouble finding relief from one of these top natural remedies, please consider visiting the website to dig deeper into the wisdom that only our readers' personal experiences can provide!

Abdominal Pain

Abdominal pain - sharp or dull, chronic or passing - can be a symptom of more critical conditions. Common causes include gas/flatulence, indigestion, and gallstones but could also be a stuck ileocecal valve, pancreatitis, appendicitis, etc.

BEST REMEDY:

- **Apple Cider Vinegar:** A tablespoon taken straight can halt stomach pain due to food poisoning. Otherwise, a teaspoon to two tablespoon's worth in a large glass of water with meals can be a general tonic.

Acid Reflux

Acid Reflux or GERD is a very common condition in which the liquid content of the stomach backs up into the esophagus, causing painful burning.

BEST REMEDIES:

- **Apple Cider Vinegar:** A teaspoon to two tablespoon's worth in a large glass of water with meals can balance the stomach's acid content and prevent acid reflux.
- **Apple Cider Vinegar and Baking Soda:** One-quarter teaspoon of baking soda with up to two tablespoons of apple cider vinegar in a large glass of water can balance the stomach's acid content and prevent acid reflux.
- **Pickle Juice:** Stop a bad acid reflux attack by drinking up to a half cup of pickle juice.
- **Dietary Changes:** Some dietary changes such as having several small meals throughout the day, avoiding fatty foods or carbs, and eliminating sodas can reduce acid reflux symptoms.

- **Apples:** An apple (or two) a day is reported to prevent acid reflux and can be used to stop an attack. Applesauce and apple juice can sometimes work as well.
- **Aloe Vera:** A bit of aloe juice straight from the leaf, commercial aloe vera juice, or aloe vera gel caps can be taken with meals to soothe the throat and stomach.
- **Digestive Enzymes:** Health stores offer tablets containing "digestive enzymes" that can be taken with meals.
- **Baking Soda:** 1/8 - 1/2 teaspoon of baking soda in a glass of water can halt the pain of acid reflux.
- **Lemons:** Real lemonade or a squeeze of lemon in a glass of water with your meal can prevent GERD symptoms.
- **Licorice Root Extract:** DGL or "Deglycyrrhizinated" Licorice Root Extract is available from health stores. Two pills a day is said to cure acid reflux.
- **Acidophilus:** This probiotic commonly found in yogurt can also be taken in pill form.
- **Betaine Hydrochloride:** Betaine HCL is available in capsule form. It effectively adds hydrochloric acid to your stomach, improving digestion to stop the attacks.
- **Mustard:** A teaspoonful or two of mustard can stop the symptoms of an acid reflux attack in its tracks.

Acne

Common acne is generally most acute in teenagers but can still be an occasional or constant problem for adults as well. The face, back, and chest are most commonly affected.

BEST REMEDIES:
- **Apple Cider Vinegar:** A daily ACV tonic (1 tsp - 2 Tbsp apple cider vinegar in a large glass of water, w/ or w/o honey) can clarify the skin and give it a healthy glow. A couple of teaspoons of ACV diluted in a cup of water can be used as a skin toner.
- **Hydrogen Peroxide:** Dip a cotton ball in hydrogen peroxide, then dab it all over the affected skin. Hold the

cotton ball to existing blemishes for a couple of minutes for deeper treatment.

- **Coconut Oil:** Using coconut oil as a daily moisturizer on the affected areas of the skin can clear up breakouts and improve the overall look of your skin.
- **Tea Tree Oil:** Use a cotton swab to dab tea tree oil on existing acne a few times a day to dry out the oily skin and clear up the blemish.
- **Garlic:** Add raw garlic to your daily diet and its antibacterial allicin compound will kill off the bacteria that cause acne on your skin.
- **Lemons:** Use a bit of lemon juice like a toner to clear away excess oils and clarify your skin. Feel free to dilute in a bit of water as well if the lemon has a bit of a bite to it.
- **Baking Soda:** Make a paste of a bit of baking soda and water, then use as a facial scrub. For more extensive body acne, put two tablespoons of baking soda in your bathwater.
- **Aloe Vera:** Apply aloe vera gel directly to your skin 2-3 times a day to clean and dry up excess oils on your skin.

Acne Scars

Even after the acne has cleared up, acne scars can last for years and be an unsightly frustration.

BEST REMEDY:
- **Aloe Vera:** The antibacterial and anti-inflammatory properties of pure (especially fresh) aloe vera gel, when rubbed into acne scars 2-3 times a day, can reduce and eliminate their appearance. It may reduce the occurrence of breakouts too!

Allergies

Hay fever and seasonal allergies can be an annual nightmare for some of us, but a few natural remedies can prevent allergy attacks or at least reduce allergic symptoms.

BEST REMEDIES:
- **Apple Cider Vinegar:** A bit of apple cider vinegar in a tall glass of water once a day can stop an allergy attack and reduce seasonal allergy symptoms. Start with one teaspoon and built up to as much as two tablespoons. You can add a touch of raw local honey as well for added effect.
- **Turmeric:** It's not exactly a spoonful of sugar, but a teaspoon of turmeric powder in a glass of water can stop a dripping nose and sore throat due to allergies. Turmeric in capsule form is also available from health food stores.
- **Honey:** Enjoying some raw local honey (or chewing honeycomb) before the start of allergy season can give your body a sort of vaccination to prevent or reduce seasonal allergy symptoms. Try one teaspoon at bedtime to combat allergies and help you sleep better as well!

Anemia

Anemia is actually a shortage of hemoglobin in the body - the protein that helps carry oxygen in the blood - but we most often think of it as a shortage of iron, since it is that lack of iron that reduces the amount of hemoglobin in an anemic person, causing fatigue and other symptoms.

BEST REMEDY:
- **Blackstrap Molasses:** Add a tablespoon of blackstrap molasses to your diet each day, and that single serving can supply 70% of your daily iron needs. Look for blackstrap (and possibly unsulphured) molasses. It may only be available in a health food store, but it will be richer than the ordinary sort you find in grocery stores.

Anxiety

The constant, almost inexplicable uneasiness of anxiety is fairly epidemic these days and can take a real toll on your general health and sense of well being, a genuine dis-ease.

BEST REMEDIES:
- **Cold Showers:** End your daily shower with a cold-water rinse for a minute or so. Be sure to target the head and lymph nodes (armpits, neck, groin, etc.). Great for fighting depression and boosting energy too!
- **Rhodiola:** Rhodiola rosea is a flowering plant in the same family as the Jade Plant. Available in pill form, its active components offer many people almost instant relief from anxiety and depression.
- **Apple Cider Vinegar:** The familiar apple cider vinegar tonic (1tsp-2 Tbsp ACV in a tall glass of water, natural sweetener optional) can balance the body in a way that seems to quickly reduce anxiety symptoms, including high blood pressure.

Arthritis

The inflammation and pain of osteoarthritis and rheumatoid arthritis can be debilitating. Natural measures to protect and restore cartilage and bone at the joints can help.

BEST REMEDIES:
- **Apple Cider Vinegar:** Easily our most popular remedy for arthritis. Some people experience remarkable transformations with continued use! Try sipping this ACV tonic throughout the day—32oz. of water, up to a quarter-cup of unpasteurized apple cider vinegar (start with a tablespoon), and optional natural sweetener.
- **Turmeric:** The Indian spice turmeric is a wondrous anti-inflammatory with a variety of medical benefits, including the reduction of arthritis pain and inflammation. Turmeric pills are available, or try a teaspoonful mixed in a glass of warm milk (almond or rice will do as well as dairy).
- **Blackstrap Molasses:** The many minerals available in large quantities in blackstrap molasses (not the typical stuff from the grocery store) could be the reason many people have found relief from arthritis pain with a daily tablespoon of blackstrap molasses.

Asthma

Chronic asthma symptoms can be not only disruptive but also disturbing and occasionally life threatening. Finding a natural way to prevent asthma attacks can reduce the strain on your body.

BEST REMEDIES:
- **Apple Cider Vinegar:** The apple cider vinegar tonic has helped some people entirely give up their inhalers! Most asthma suffers choose two tablespoonfuls in a large glass of water (honey or other natural sweetener optional), but you can start with a smaller amount of vinegar if you like. Really clears congestion.
- **Dietary Changes:** Eliminating dairy or choosing an alkaline diet might be the simple secret to eliminating your asthma condition.
- **Coffee:** A hot cup of black coffee can offer quick relief from an asthma attack, between the steamy cup and coffee's ability to stimulate the body.

Athlete's Foot

Common Athlete's Foot (also jock itch) is a fungal infection that causes an irritating rash, itching, broken skin, and redness on the skin. The infection can be passed casually from infected surfaces and often shows up between the toes and on the feet.

BEST REMEDIES:
- **Apple Cider Vinegar:** Applied directly to the infected skin, apple cider vinegar can kill off the fungus that causes the infection while disinfecting the foot. Unlike other vinegars (which will also kill the fungus), apple cider vinegar will also soothe the burning feeling. Dab on the affected area or soak feet in a warm water bath with a cup of apple cider vinegar for half an hour. Be warned though, it might burn a bit worse on contact!
- **Urine:** Odd but true! Simply urinating on your own feet while in the shower can kill off the athlete's foot

fungus. Wash the urine off as the last thing you do in the shower so that it has time to take effect.

B

Bad Breath

Halitosis, or good old bad breath, is a common problem with no end of commercial "solutions". Dental, digestive, and infectious conditions can be the root cause.

BEST REMEDY:
- **Hydrogen Peroxide:** An occasional mouthwash that is 1 part 3% hydrogen peroxide to 5 parts water can instantly and lastingly cure bad breath. HP real gets rid of all those bad breath bacteria!

Back Pain

Acute and chronic back pain conditions can have a number of causes, from muscle damage to nerve issues.

BEST REMEDIES:
- **Apple Cider Vinegar:** A twice-daily ACV tonic (1tsp-2Tbsp apple cider vinegar in a large glass of water—natural sweetener optional) can rebalance your mineral supply and revitalize the body as a whole.
- **Coconut Oil:** Rubbing a bit of coconut oil into the affected area of your back can relieve back pain within minutes. It's great for the skin too!

Bacterial Vaginosis

An imbalance in the body's natural variety and amount of bacteria results in bacterial vaginosis, the most common type of bacterial infection. An unpleasant "fishy" smell and off-white vaginal discharge are the primary symptoms.

BEST REMEDIES:

- **Hydrogen Peroxide:** 3% hydrogen peroxide, usually mixed with equal parts water, can be used as a douche or applied to a tampon (for temporary use, maybe 20-30 minutes).
- **Acidophilus:** Acidophilus pills can be taken orally and inserted vaginally to add healthy bacteria to the vagina and restore your balance.
- **Folic Acid:** 800 mcg of folic acid taken orally on a daily basis seems to strengthen the body and restore balance to the vaginal environment so that the smell and discharge go away. The CDC recommends at least 400mcg daily for all women, regardless.
- **Boric Acid:** A capsule of boric acid inserted into the vagina can quickly stop the smell and discharge. Finding boric acid can be tricky, but your pharmacist should be able to order it for you.
- **Probiotics:** Probiotic pills (they should be refrigerated!) are available that specifically target BV and similar conditions. Not all probiotics will have the same effect, so take your time in finding the right probiotic mix.
- **Yogurt:** Plain yogurt with live cultures can be eaten or applied directly (try filling a tampon applicator) to restore your supply of healthy bacteria and stop the odor and discharge.

Bee Stings

The pain of a bee sting can be lasting and extreme, but a few natural remedies can reduce the bee's bite! Of course, anyone allergic to bee stings should always have an epi-pen available.

BEST REMEDIES:

- **Apple Cider Vinegar:** Soak a cotton ball in apple cider vinegar and apply it directly to the bee sting for several minutes. The acid will neutralize the sting's toxin, stopping the pain and reducing any redness or swelling.

- **Tobacco:** Your grandpa will tell you—moisten and place a bit of tobacco leaf on any bee sting to stop the pain and swelling within minutes!

Bladder Infections

A bladder infection, or more generally a urinary tract infection (UTI), results when bacteria get into the bladder or kidneys and multiply. The pain and discomfort can be remedied at home, but serious or reoccurring pain should be addressed with a doctor.

BEST REMEDIES:
- **Apple Cider Vinegar:** A day or two of twice daily ACV tonics should halt a bladder infection, but continue for a few days afterward to make sure—take 1-2 tablespoons apple cider vinegar, unsweetened, in a tall glass of water.
- **Cranberry:** Cranberry pills and unsweetened cranberry juice can put an end to bladder infections.
- **D-Mannose:** D-mannose seems to be the active ingredient in cranberry juice that prevents and may stop a bladder infection. You can find D-mannose pills at some health food stores and pharmacies.
- **Alka Seltzer:** Take Alka Seltzer as directed to relieve bladder infection symptoms quickly. May not kill off the infection, but the relief is well worth it!
- **Apple Cider Vinegar and Baking Soda:** Two or three times a day, drink a large glass of water with 1-2 tablespoons of apple cider vinegar and an eighth of a teaspoon of baking soda (watch out for the fizz!).
- **Baking Soda:** Half a teaspoon of baking soda dissolved in a glass of water 2-3 times a day can provide instant relief from the burning. It will eventually remedy a bladder infection by restoring an alkaline balance to your body.
- **Sea Salt:** A one-dose remedy (and no more than once!). Add a teaspoon of sea salt to a large glass of water and drink. Very effective, especially if combined with other UTI remedies.

Bloating

Bloating and fluid retention can be uncomfortable and make it tough to get into our favorite clothes! It's usually a sign of some imbalance in the body.

BEST REMEDY:
- **Apple Cider Vinegar:** A daily ACV tonic can restore your body's mineral balance and reduce bloating. Start with one teaspoon of apple cider vinegar in a tall glass of water and build up to as much as two tablespoons. Take a few days off the tonic every so often.

Blood Pressure

High blood pressure (above 120/80), known as hypertension, is a critical health concern that can lead to heart conditions, stroke, and other significant health concerns.

BEST REMEDIES:
- **Apple Cider Vinegar:** Taking the ACV tonic 2-3 times a day can significantly lower your blood pressure. Start with one teaspoon of apple cider vinegar in a large glass of water and build up to one or two tablespoons. Add honey or other natural sweetener for taste.
- **Cayenne Pepper:** Cayenne pepper pills are available, but simply adding a teaspoon of cayenne to your daily meals can significantly reduce blood pressure almost immediately. Try adding it to hot water for an invigorating beverage!
- **Garlic:** A clove of raw garlic each day (or garlic tablets) can lower blood pressure effectively. Try a bit of fennel or parsley to block the garlic breath afterwards!
- **Apple Cider Vinegar and Baking Soda:** Add an eighth of a teaspoon of baking soda to the standard ACV tonic (two teaspoons of apple cider vinegar in a large glass of water) for a blood pressure remedy that is even more effective for some people than the straight tonic.

Blood Sugar

While our bodies run largely on sugar, high (hyperglycemia) or low (hypoglycemia) blood sugar can be a real problem. Diabetes is the greatest concern for continued hyperglycemia.

BEST REMEDY:

- **Apple Cider Vinegar:** A daily (or up to thrice daily) ACV tonic can steady the rate of digestion, lengthening the amount of time the body has to process new sugars and keeping blood sugar levels more even. Start with one teaspoon of apple cider vinegar in a tall glass of water with meals, and increase the dose to as much as 2 tablespoons per glass.

Body Odor

While sweat itself has very little odor, it can promote the growth of bacteria on the skin, and these bacteria can have strong odors. Diet, bathing, health, medications, and other factors can influence body odor.

BEST REMEDIES:

- **Baking Soda:** The ultimate odor absorber, baking soda can eliminate body odor as well. If you would like to avoid commercial deodorants, try mixing baking soda in a bit of body lotion or mixing 2 Tbsp in a cup of water that you can apply to your underarms with a spray bottle. Or just apply a bit directly to the skin!
- **Apple Cider Vinegar:** Use a cotton swab to apply apple cider vinegar directly to the affected skin. Leave on for a couple of minutes, then wash off. The vinegar will kill the offensive bacteria and improve the health of your skin as well!
- **Milk of Magnesia:** An unlikely remedy, but one with enthusiastic supporters! Just rub a bit of MoM under your arms as a deodorant and allow to dry. No more odor!
- **Avoid Caffeine:** Cutting coffee, tea, and caffeinated

sodas out of your diet (or at least drastically reducing your caffeine intake) can have a remarkable effect on body odor.

Body Rash

A rash can take on any number of appearances and annoying characteristics - from the merely unsightly to the downright aggravating - and can be caused by a wide variety of infections, allergens, or wider medical conditions.

BEST REMEDIES:
- **Apple Cider Vinegar:** Dabbing undiluted apple cider vinegar on a rash can relieve itching and irritation quickly. The nutrients in unpasteurized ACV can also help to heal the skin while the acetic acid kills off possible infections or even the agent causing the rash. Apply for a few minutes several times a day.
- **Coconut Oil:** Rub a bit of natural coconut oil into a rash - just like body lotion - and experience quick relief from irritation. Often the rash soon disappears as well. Great for diaper rash!

Boils

Boils seem to be increasingly common. Usually the result of a staph infection, this form of folliculitis results in an accumulation of pus and a hard core at the center of the boil that will need to be removed.

BEST REMEDIES:
- **Turmeric:** Far and away the most popular boil remedy, turmeric is a powerful health aid (and a spice) from India. Drink one teaspoon of turmeric in water 2-3 times a day until the boil has healed.
- **Baking Soda:** A paste of baking soda and water can be applied to a boil and left on to draw out the infection and dry out the boil.

- **Garlic:** Eating a clove of raw garlic daily can help kill a staph infection from the inside. You can also crush the garlic into a paste and apply it to a boil for 10-20 minutes at a time, 2-3 times a day.
- **Iodine:** Apply povidone iodine to a boil and the area immediately around it to stop a boil and prevent the staph infection from spreading.
- **Apple Cider Vinegar:** Dab a cotton ball in apple cider vinegar and tape it to the boil, then replace it twice a day. Also, try the ACV tonic (1tsp-2Tbsp apple cider vinegar in a tall glass of water, natural sweetener optional).

Bronchitis

The inflammation of the airways that characterizes bronchitis will be accompanied by coughing and phlegm production. Wheezing and shortness of breath are also common.

BEST REMEDIES:
- **Apple Cider Vinegar:** Stop the cough, reduce the phlegm, and kill off the virus or bacteria causing your bronchitis with an ACV tonic of 1 tablespoon apple cider vinegar and two teaspoons honey mixed in a warm, tall glass of water.
- **Garlic:** A clove or two of raw garlic added to your daily diet can clean the bronchitis-causing pathogen out of your body and cut through your congestion.

Burns

A mild-to-moderate burn can be treated at home with natural remedies to prevent infection of the affected skin. The best remedies reduce pain and swelling almost immediately.

BEST REMEDIES:
- **Egg Whites:** Separate egg whites into a bowl and soak the affected body part in the egg whites, or apply egg

whites directly to the skin and allow to dry. This most popular burn remedy can immediately relieve the pain of a burn, and after a few hours application, you may find that there is no remaining sign or symptom from even a significant burn.

- **Aluminum Foil:** Apply the shiny side of aluminum foil to a burn and be amazed! The pain may increase briefly, but then should subside and may be completely gone within half an hour.
- **Baking Soda:** Make a paste of baking soda and water, then apply it to the burn. When it dries and pain returns, rinse and reapply.
- **Vinegar:** Soak a cotton ball in vinegar and apply to the burn (or use it to dab vinegar all over a sunburn) to experience quick relief. Kills potential pathogens that could infect an open blister as well.
- **Honey:** Apply honey directly to a burn—the pain vanishes immediately! Honey has antibiotic properties that help prevent infection as well.
- **Mustard:** Apply mustard to a burn, then rinse and reapply when it dries off and any pain returns. You can also wrap the burned area in gauze to prevent staining from the mustard.
- **Toothpaste:** Spread a good coating of toothpaste on a burn and expect relief within a few minutes. Any brand should do, but a mint flavor is most likely to bring relief!

Bursitis

As likely as not, you were hardly aware that you had bursae - little fluid-filled sacs that allow smooth movement between muscles, tendons, and the like - but when they become inflamed with bursitis, every movement announces their presence.

BEST REMEDY:
- **Apple Cider Vinegar:** Take one teaspoon of apple cider vinegar (ACV) with one teaspoon of (raw) honey

in a tall glass of water and drink 2-3 times a day. You can eventually increase the amount of ACV up to as much as two tablespoons. Try soaking a cloth in ACV as well and binding it to the afflicted area.

C

Cancer

The uncontrolled growth of cells is the one thing that unites all of the many forms of cancer, whether that cancer involves a tumor(s), metastasizes, is malignant or benign.

BEST REMEDIES:

- **Budwig Diet:** While many changes in diet and habits can help prevent cancer or improve cancer symptoms, according to the Earth Clinic community, so far only the Budwig Diet (from Nobel Prize winner Dr. Johanna Budwig) seems to have the potential to turn back cancerous growths. Please search Earth Clinic or another reliable source for the diet's exact details.
- **Ted's Cancer Regimen:** Our in-house expert Ted has extensive theories on how to address multiple forms of cancer. A few points are universal to these treatments: 1) eliminate sugars (especially fructose), 2) supplement with 1/2 teaspoon lysine and 1/2 teaspoon n-acetyl cysteine every hour for at least 4 hours over three days, 3) take 1/8 teaspoon of tannic acid and/or 1/4 teaspoon green tea extract three times a day, plus 4) 1000 mg sodium ascorbate (Vitamin C) 8 times a day for the first three days. After those first three days, the supplements can be taken in much reduced quantities.

Candida

Our high-sugar diets can allow Candida yeasts to grow out of control in our bodies, creating infections called thrush or candidiasis. This fungal infection can strike almost anywhere in the body and have a variety of negative effects.

BEST REMEDY:

- **Hydrogen Peroxide:** The cleansing ability of hydrogen peroxide can kill off the excess candida cells and stop the fungal infection. Very careful use of 35% Food Grade hydrogen peroxide - starting with just one drop in a large glass of distilled water - can kill off a case of candidiasis. Take three glasses a day, not around meal times, with the number of drops slowly growing to as many as 10 drops per glass.
- **Acidophilus:** Taking acidophilus capsules daily can substantially increase your body's own ability to restore its homeostasis and drive out the candida overgrowth. Be sure to find a supplement that guarantees more than 2 billion live cells per capsule, and use as directed.

Canker Sores

The painful oral ulcers of a canker sore outbreak can be an isolated sore or coat the throat and mouth in open sores. While not contagious, the root cause of a canker sore is unknown.

BEST REMEDIES:

- **Apple Cider Vinegar:** For immediate relief, apply apple cider vinegar (ACV) directly to a canker sore. For long-term freedom from sores, try a daily ACV tonic—one teaspoon of ACV in a large glass of water. Increase the dose of ACV up to as much as two tablespoons, according to your body's needs.
- **Aspirin:** Apply an aspirin tablet directly to a canker sore and hold for 5-10 minutes twice a day. The pain will soon disappear, eventually along with the sore. For multiple sores, try crushing a tablet in a glass of water and holding the water in your mouth. Spit out afterwards (you don't want to swallow the canker toxins).
- **Alum:** Alum, which can be found in the spice rack of your grocery store, can be briefly applied to a canker sore 2-3 times a day to get rid of sores. It will hurt, and

you will want to wash the bad taste out of your mouth, but it can be very effective.

- **Baking Soda:** Make a paste of baking soda and water, and then apply it to any canker sore. Leave it be for as long as possible. Reapply a few times a day and expect to be rid of the sore within a few days.
- **Salt:** If you can tolerate the brief increase in pain, a bit of salt dabbed on a canker sore or a warm saltwater mouthwash can get rid of a canker sore in a few applications.
- **Hydrogen Peroxide:** Dab a bit of hydrogen peroxide on a canker sore, or use a small bit of hydrogen peroxide as a mouthwash, to kill off whatever infection is creating the sores.
- **L-Lysine:** L-Lysine tablets taken twice a day can cure an attack of canker sores. Supplementing this essential amino acid seems to restore the body's ability to heal itself.
- **Toothpaste w/o SLS:** The abrasive nature of brushing your teeth can trigger a canker sore on its own. Worse yet, SLS (Sodium Lauryl Sulfite), is a common preservative that seems to be a further trigger. So be certain to choose a toothpaste free of SLS and you might stop your canker sore attacks.
- **Yogurt:** The active cultures in yogurt may be able to restore balance to the internal chemistry of your mouth, throat, and overall digestive system and thereby cure the canker sores. Simply eat yogurt containing active cultures once or twice a day.

Cellulite

Cellulite, the uneven appearance of skin around the legs, hips, and abdomen of adults is, in fact, common to most women but nonetheless considered unsightly and unwanted.

BEST REMEDY:

- **Coconut Oil:** Extra Virgin Coconut Oil can be an excellent all-around health and beauty aid. To treat cellulite, use the coconut oil directly on the skin as a moisturizer. Many also add it to their diet for a number of positive effects. Start with ¼ teaspoon daily. You can slowly work up to a daily tablespoon's worth.

Cholesterol

Cholesterol is simply a type of fat (a lipid) found in many foods. High cholesterol levels in the body and bloodstream, however, can result in clogged arteries (atherosclerosis), contributing to heart disease and the possibility of a heart attack or stroke.

BEST REMEDIES:

- **Apple Cider Vinegar:** To lower your overall cholesterol levels in short time, take the Apple Cider Vinegar tonic 2-3 times daily with meals. Start with one teaspoon apple cider vinegar in a tall glass of water (natural sweetener optional), and slowly increase the amount of vinegar to as much as 2 tablespoons per glass according to your body's needs.
- **Red Yeast Rice:** Red yeast rice is the newest discovery in natural cholesterol treatment. Available in tablets, take as directed.
- **Coconut Oil:** It may seem counterintuitive to add an oil to your diet to lower cholesterol, but many have been able to lower their LDLs with just the addition of Extra Virgin Coconut Oil to their diet. Start with ¼ teaspoon a day and slowly increase to as much as a daily tablespoon.

Coating on Tongue

A white coating on the tongue may just be dead skin cells, but if it cannot be easily brushed off with a toothbrush, it may be thrush and most likely caused by a Candida infection.

BEST REMEDIES:
- **Oil Pulling:** The ancient practice of oil pulling is finding renewed fame for its ability to pull toxins out of the body. Before brushing your teeth and with an empty stomach, take one Tbsp of oil into your mouth and swish it around for 10-20 minutes until the oil has turned milky white. Then spit out. Most any food oil can do, but sesame and sunflower oils are traditional and the most popular.
- **Salt:** Take sea salt or kosher salt and use salt water as a mouthwash. For tough cases, follow up by placing salt directly on the tongue and holding it there for a few minutes before spitting out. Or put salt on your toothbrush and brush your tongue with it.

Colds

Ah, the common cold. The illness that launched a thousand remedies, but which natural remedy really puts a stop to the sniffles, sneezing, congestion, and runny, stuffed up nose?

BEST REMEDIES:
- **Jean's Famous Tomato Tea:** Outrageously popular, this simple home remedy from our friend Jeannie Woolhiser of Wisconsin clears sinus congestion almost immediately and can bring a quick end to a cold. Mix and heat the following recipe on the stove, then drink and inhale the steam (be careful!) until after your symptoms have disappeared.

  TOMATO TEA RECIPE
  2 cups tomato juice
  2-3 cloves garlic crushed (use more if you can)
  2 T lemon juice
  Hot sauce (the more the better, so as much as you can handle)

- **Apple Cider Vinegar:** Take a tablespoon each of apple cider vinegar and honey in a warm but not hot glass of water up to three times a day to relieve all cold symptoms, including sore throat.
- **Garlic:** The sulfur in raw garlic seems to make it a strong antiviral/antibacterial remedy. Add a clove of raw garlic to your food 3-4 times a day to combat all cold symptoms and bring a cold to a quick conclusion.
- **Cayenne Pepper:** Add a teaspoon of cayenne pepper to a glass of water or a bowl of soup to completely clear the sinuses, cure a sore throat, and speed to the end of a cold. Repeat daily, up to three times a day.
- **Hydrogen Peroxide:** At the first sign of a cold, lie on your side and put a few drops of hydrogen peroxide in your ear, and then let it sit for several minutes. Then empty out that ear and repeat on the other side. Hydrogen peroxide's antiviral properties seem to cut the cold virus down before it can take hold.
- **Vitamin C:** Take about 1000 mg of Vitamin C as soon as you feel a cold coming on and you can halt or reduce the cold symptoms dramatically. Repeat 2-3 times a day and continue to take Vitamin C for as long as the cold continues.
- **Oil of Oregano:** A drop of oil of oregano under the tongue, or one to three drops in a glass of water, can encourage expectoration and help clear the throat, nose, and lungs of congestion.

Cold Sores

Cold sores, caused by the herpes simplex virus, are fairly common but nonetheless irritating and embarrassing. We have found that they are triggered and exacerbated by artificial sweeteners. Yet one more reason to avoid them!

BEST REMEDIES:
- **Acetone Nail Polish Remover:** Use a cotton swab to

apply a bit of acetone nail polish remover to a cold sore about once an hour until the cold sore is gone—often in a day or two!

- **Hydrogen Peroxide:** Dip a cotton swab in hydrogen peroxide and apply to any cold sore every few hours throughout the day to get rid of a cold sore within about three days.

- **Apple Cider Vinegar:** You'll feel a bit of a burning at first, but if you dab a bit of apple cider vinegar on a cold sore, it should dry out and disappear within about three days. Reapply about 4-5 times a day.

- **Ear Wax:** Odd but true! As soon as you get a cold sore tingle, apply a bit of your own ear wax to the spot to stop the eruption from ever forming. Works even after the cold sore has formed. Leave it on, but don't lick your lips (yuck!).

- **L-Lysine:** Start taking the essential amino acid L-Lysine (in pill form) as soon as you feel a cold sore forming. You can reduce the number/size of cold stores or stop the outbreak entirely.

- **Garlic:** Cut a clove of garlic in small pieces and hold a piece to your cold sore for about ten minutes, 3-5 times a day (no more!) to dry out your cold sore and kill the virus at the same time.

- **Coconut Oil:** Adding up to a tablespoonful of cold pressed coconut oil to your daily diet (start with an eighth of a teaspoonful and increase slowly) can put an end to your cold sore attacks. For an active cold sore, try applying coconut oil directly to the sore a few times a day and leaving it there.

Congestion

Sinus congestion and congestion in the throat and lungs can be debilitating and even dangerous. Mucus/phlegm plays a role in preventing illness, but too much of it can be just as much of a problem, not to mention the discomfort.

BEST REMEDIES:

- **Jean's Famous Tomato Tea:** Outrageously popular, this simple home remedy from our friend Jeannie Woolhiser of Wisconsin clears sinus congestion almost immediately and can bring a quick end to a cold. Mix and heat the following recipe on the stove, then drink and inhale the steam (be careful!) until after your symptoms have disappeared.

  ### TOMATO TEA RECIPE
  2 cups tomato juice
  2-3 cloves garlic crushed (use more if you can)
  2 T lemon juice
  Hot sauce (the more the better, so as much as you can handle)

- **Apple Cider Vinegar:** The apple cider vinegar tonic, taken two-three times a day, can quickly break up congestion and improve other cold and flu symptoms as well. Add one tablespoon each apple cider vinegar and honey to a tall glass of warm water, and sip.
- **Oil Pulling:** The Ayurvedic tradition of oil pulling can remove toxins from the body and clear up congestion as well. Before brushing your teeth and with an empty stomach, take one Tbsp of oil into your mouth and swish it around for 10-20 minutes until the oil has turned milky white. Then spit out. Most any food oil will do, but sesame and sunflower oils are traditional and the most popular.
- **Neti Pot:** The traditional neti pot can be an excellent general health tool, but it is especially effective at cleaning out the sinuses and relieving congestion. Check out EarthClinic.com or a trusted source on the proper use of neti pots.
- **Steaming:** Drape a towel over your head and neck, then carefully hold your face over a steaming pot of water (not too hot!). Breathe in the steam for several minutes, and repeat throughout the day. For added effect, try adding

lavender oil, a tablespoon of apple cider vinegar, or some essential oils from the mint family for even greater effect.

Conjunctivitis

Conjunctivitis is better known as 'pink eye', and is a viral infection that causes irritation, watering, reddening of the eyes, and a distinct pinkness to the eye's conjunctiva (the combined area at the edge of the eye and on the inside of the eyelid). A bacterial form is also possible.

BEST REMEDIES:
- **Apple Cider Vinegar:** Mix about two teaspoons of unpasteurized apple cider vinegar in a cup of water, then dip a cotton pad or soft cloth in it to wash the eyelid inside and out. You can place a few drops of the water mixture in the eye as well. Repeat every few hours until the conjunctivitis is all gone, usually 2-3 days.
- **Green Tea Bags:** Put two green tea bags in a cup of hot water and allow the tea to brew and then cool somewhat, then apply each bag to an eye. Rewarm in the water and continue for about 10 minutes. Repeat every few hours until healed, usually 2-3 days.
- **Colloidal Silver:** Place a drop of colloidal silver in the affected eye 2-3 times a day until symptoms are gone.
- **Sea Salt:** Combine a tablespoon of sea salt in a cup of water and apply 2-3 drops to the corners of your eyes first thing in the morning and last thing at night.
- **Black Tea Bag:** Make a cup of black tea and allow it to cool a bit. Then apply the tea bag to the eye and keep it there for ten minutes or so. Repeat every few hours for the 1-3 days it will take to clear up the conjunctivitis.

COPD

Chronic Obstructive Pulmonary Disease (COPD) is a set of conditions including emphysema and bronchitis that obstructs airflow to and from the lungs. Smoking is the most frequent cause, and a complete cure is rare.

BEST REMEDY:

- **Hydrogen Peroxide Inhalation:** While it should be undertaken carefully, using an emptied nasal spray bottle to inhale 3% hydrogen peroxide can open up airways and reduce COPD symptoms. (Be sure to first sterilize the spray bottle with boiling water.) Point the spray bottle in your mouth and at the back of your throat, and while inhaling sharply pump 4-6 sprays of the hydrogen peroxide. Repeat 4-6 times a day.

Constipation

Constipation is a common digestive system problem in which one experiences infrequent bowel movements, hard stools, or straining during bowel movements. The general rule of thumb is that if you are passing hard and dry stools less than three times a week, you probably have constipation.

BEST REMEDIES:

- **Apple Cider Vinegar:** The apple cider vinegar (ACV) tonic is easily our most popular remedy for all manner of complaints. Start with one teaspoon apple cider vinegar and an equal amount of honey in a tall glass of water. Later on, slowly increase the amount of vinegar to as much as 2 tablespoons per glass according to your body's needs. Take 2-3 times daily with meals.
- **Magnesium:** Adding magnesium supplements to your diet might be all it takes for regular, pain-free bowel movements.
- **Molasses:** Many people have had success in adding one tablespoon of blackstrap molasses (a more concentrated form than most grocery store brands) twice a day to their diets. The concentrated minerals in the molasses seem to do the trick.
- **Lemon Juice and Olive Oil:** To quickly relieve

constipation, try mixing one Tbsp of olive oil together with one Tbsp of lemon juice, and drink. Take 2-3 times a day, but only while experiencing constipation.

Coughs

A cough is meant to rid the body of antigens, viruses, and bacteria to prevent or bring an end to an infection. However, too much coughing can just be irritating and counterproductive.

BEST REMEDIES:
- **Apple Cider Vinegar:** The apple cider vinegar tonic, taken two-three times a day, can quickly break up congestion and soothe a cough. Add one tablespoon each apple cider vinegar and honey to a tall glass of warm water, and sip.
- **Onions:** Cut an onion in half and cover each half of the cut with honey, brown sugar, or another sugar and set aside for an hour. A syrup will form that should be taken like cough syrup as needed until your cough subsides.
- **Garlic:** Add a clove of raw garlic to your food or eat/chew it directly if you can stand it. Try 1-2 cloves a day until your cough goes away.

Cradle Cap

Although it does not bother most babies and is very common, the crusty, yellowish rash called cradle cap can be unsightly on a newborn baby.

BEST REMEDY:
- **Baking Soda Paste:** Mix baking soda together with enough water to form a paste and gently rub into the baby's scalp. Rinse off immediately and repeat once a day until the cradle cap disappears, usually within a few days.

Cuts

Cuts or lacerations to the skin are common enough, but should be treated with care. Any wound, no matter how small, can become infected and lead to more significant health problems.

BEST REMEDY:
- **Cayenne:** Powdered cayenne pepper can rapidly staunch blood flow and help a wound heal much faster. You can leave the cayenne on and cover with a bandage.

Cystic Acne

While not entirely uncommon, cystic acne can be very uncomfortable. Acne cysts form much like ordinary pimples, from an excess of sebum, but in this case the pus forms into small cysts.

BEST REMEDY:
- **Turmeric:** Add a teaspoon of the spice turmeric to a small glass of milk (almond or rice will do as well as dairy), add honey if you like, and drink twice a day to clear up cystic acne almost overnight!

Dandruff

The itchy scalp of a dandruff condition and the embarrassing white flakes compete to see which can be the worse symptom of this common condition.

BEST REMEDIES:
- **Apple Cider Vinegar:** Dilute apple cider vinegar 1:1 with water and then use just like a shampoo to clean your hair and scalp. Should cure the itch instantly and get rid of dandruff within several days worth of applications.
- **Apple Cider Vinegar and Hydrogen Peroxide:** Combine 1 part apple cider vinegar and 1 part Hydrogen Peroxide with 10 parts water. Use like a shampoo and rinse after the mixture has set for a few minutes. Should clear up dandruff in 2-3 days.
- **Omega 3 Supplements:** Fish oil or flaxseed oil will provide your body with needed omega 3 fatty acids. Along with a host of other benefits, these omega 3's can improve scalp nutrition and hydration. Just be careful that you get pharmaceutical grade fish oil if you choose fish over flaxseed, so as to avoid mercury and other heavy metal contaminants.

Deep Vein Thrombosis

An inflamed vein, called phlebitis, can be extremely uncomfortable. It can be associated with Deep Vein Thrombosis, otherwise known as 'economy class syndrome'.

BEST REMEDY:
- **Ted's Lemon and Baking Soda Remedy:** Take the freshly squeezed juice of a lemon (or lime) and slowly add

baking soda to the glass until the mixture stops fizzing, then add 4 oz. of water. Take twice a day, once in the morning and once before bedtime on an empty stomach.

Depression

Depression can be a simple period of sadness or negativity, but it can also be an uncontrollable and enduring hopeless or gloomy mood. It may be accompanied by physical symptoms as well, and at its worst can lead to thoughts of or attempts at suicide.

BEST REMEDIES:

- **Cold Showers:** A simple cold shower can stimulate the immune system and pleasure-producing neurotransmitters in the brain for a quick and lasting change in mood. If you can't handle an entire cold shower, start by turning the hot water down to as cold as you can get it for a couple of minutes, dousing your head and lymph nodes.
- **Apple Cider Vinegar:** The apple cider vinegar (ACV) tonic is easily our most popular remedy for all manner of complaints. Start with one-teaspoon apple cider vinegar and an equal amount of honey in a tall glass of water. Later on, slowly increase the amount of vinegar to as much as 2 tablespoons per glass according to your body's needs. Take 2-3 times daily with meals.
- **5-HTP:** 5-HTP is an amino acid that can stimulate production of serotonin in the brain. Available in pills, to be taken as directed.
- **Omega 3 Supplements:** Fish oil or flaxseed oil will provide your body with needed omega 3 fatty acids. Along with a host of other benefits, these omega 3's can substantially improve mood. Just be careful that you get pharmaceutical grade fish oil if you choose fish over flaxseed, so as to avoid mercury and other heavy metal contaminants.

Dermatitis

Dermatitis, a general inflammation of the skin, can take many forms from contact dermatitis and eczema to perioral and discoid dermatitis. It can present itself as an irritation, rash, and even blisters.

BEST REMEDIES:
- **Apple Cider Vinegar:** Apply a 50/50 concentration of apple cider vinegar and water to a rash and then rinse off after several minutes. Do this twice a day until the dermatitis heals.
- **Grapefruit Seed Extract:** Add 8-20 drops of grapefruit seed extract to 4 oz. of water and drink twice daily. You can also dab the mixture on the rash and then rinse off after a few minutes.
- **Coconut Oil:** Apply a small amount of coconut oil to any rash several times a day, just like lotion, to stop the irritation and cure most dermatitis within a few days.

Diarrhea

Any loose or liquid bowel movements are referred to as diarrhea, though it can have many causes (viral, toxic, parasites, etc.). Diarrhea that continues for many days can dehydrate the body and be very dangerous, and is in fact a major killer of young children, especially in the developing world.

BEST REMEDIES:
- **Apple Cider Vinegar:** Take 1-2 tablespoons of apple cider vinegar in a glass of water and drink. Do so twice a day until the diarrhea is completely gone (though one dose may do it for some).
- **Turmeric:** Half a teaspoon of powdered turmeric in a glass of water might be enough to stop diarrhea in one dose. Repeat several hours later if necessary.
- **Cinnamon:** Cinnamon tea can quickly cure a case of diarrhea. Break up a couple of cinnamon sticks in a

mug and pour boiling water over it, then drink. You can also add a teaspoon of powdered cinnamon to a piece of toast.

Diabetes - Type 2

Type 2 Diabetes, also known as adult-onset diabetes or non-insulin-dependent diabetes, is a chronic condition where the body cannot process sugar adequately. The resulting high blood glucose levels can cause a number of health concerns, including neuropathy and cell damage/death.

BEST REMEDY:
- **Apple Cider Vinegar:** The mix of nutrients and digestive aids in unpasteurized apple cider vinegar (ACV) can slow the digestive process and improve sugar metabolism. Take the ACV tonic three times a day with meals—one teaspoon of ACV in a large glass of water. Increase the amount of ACV to 1-2 tablespoons per glass as your body tolerates it.

Diverticulitis

Inflammation of diverticula on the colon is fairly common. Symptoms include pain (usually on the left side), fever, nausea, and changes in bowel movement patterns (diarrhea or constipation). Infection may be the cause.

BEST REMEDY:
- **Grapefruit Seed Extract:** Twelve (12) drops of grapefruit seed extract in a glass of water or orange juice twice a day can be an effective remedy for diverticulitis. After getting relief, you can begin to cut back on the dosage and frequency as your body dictates.

Dry Eyes

Dry eyes are increasingly common, with so many of us sitting in front of computers all day. It can be a congenital condition that results in reduced tear production, or may just be an environmental effect. In either case, the irritation and redness can be uncomfortable and eventually damage the eye.

BEST REMEDY:

- **Fish Oil:** Taking fish oil pills (as directed) can help your body's own self-lubricating systems take care of your eyes and end the dry eye symptoms. Just be careful that you get pharmaceutical grade fish oil, so as to avoid mercury and other heavy metal contaminants.

Dysmenorrhea

Menstrual cramps, pain, pressure, and an upset stomach can precede and accompany a woman's monthly period, in a condition called dysmenorrhea. Some cramping is normal for all women, but the additional symptoms, while common, are sometimes the result of a secondary condition.

BEST REMEDIES:

- **Blackstrap Molasses:** Add one tsp to one Tbsp of blackstrap molasses (more concentrated than the kind you'll find on most grocery store shelves). It's a strong taste, but you can combine it with many foods, and its rich mix of nutrients (and iron!) has brought many women dramatic relief.
- **Apple Cider Vinegar:** Many women have found quick relief from heavy bleeding, cramping, missed periods, and other menstruation concerns with the apple cider vinegar (ACV) tonic taken 1-3 times a day with meals. Mix 1 tsp - 2 Tbsp apple cider vinegar in a large glass of water, w/ or w/o honey, and sip slowly.

Ear Ache

Earaches can have a number of causes, some of them originating with the nose, mouth, and throat. Generally, infection is a common cause of earache.

BEST REMEDIES:

- **Hydrogen Peroxide:** For blocked or infected ears, lay a towel down on your bed or carpet. Then drip a bit of 3% hydrogen peroxide into one ear. After a few moments you will hear fizzing. Wait until the fizzing stops -- 10 to 15 minutes, occasionally adding more hydrogen peroxide. Shake remaining liquid from your ear onto the towel and repeat on the other ear.
- **Garlic:** Slice open one side of a clove of garlic to expose the interior, and cut the garlic into a piece small enough to fit into the ear but (CAUTION!) too large to slide into the ear canal. Wrap the garlic in a bit of cotton gauze or cheesecloth, and place into the opening of the ear canal.
- **Warmed Oil:** Warm up a bit of olive oil to just over body temperature and add a few drops to your ear while lying on your side. Rest for a few minutes, then pour back out. Repeat if necessary.
- **Onions:** Warm an onion to just a touch over body temperature, then squeeze some onion juice out. Add a few drops to the affected ear to quickly stop the pain. A few applications should kill the infection.

Ear Issues

Sinus pressure, ringing sounds, and pain can all bother our ears. Earaches in particular can have a number of causes, some of them originating with the nose, mouth, and throat. Generally, infection is a common cause of earache.

BEST REMEDIES:

- **Hydrogen Peroxide:** For blocked or infected ears, lay a towel down on your bed or carpet. Then drip a bit of 3% hydrogen peroxide into one ear. After a few moments you will hear fizzing. Wait until the fizzing stops -- 10 to 15 minutes, occasionally adding more hydrogen peroxide. Shake remaining liquid from your ear onto the towel and repeat on the other ear.
- **Garlic:** Slice open one side of a clove of garlic to expose the interior, and cut the garlic into a piece small enough to fit into the ear but (CAUTION!) too large to slide into the ear canal. Wrap the garlic in a bit of cotton gauze or cheesecloth, and place into the opening of the ear canal.
- **Warmed Oil:** Warm up a bit of olive oil to just over body temperature and add a few drops to your ear while lying on your side. Rest for a few minutes, then pour back out. Repeat if necessary.
- **Onions:** Warm an onion to just a touch over body temperature, then squeeze some onion juice out. Add a few drops to the affected ear to quickly stop the pain. A few applications should kill the infection.
- **Cayenne Pepper:** For ear pressure such as from a sinus headache, add one-quarter to one-half teaspoon of powdered cayenne pepper to warm water and drink. This should drain the sinuses and relieve the pressure on the ears.

Ear Wax

Earwax is an important part of our preventive immune systems, but some people produce too much of it. Sometimes too ear wax can become dry and hardened, limiting hearing.

BEST REMEDY:

- **Hydrogen Peroxide:** Lay a towel down on your bed or carpet. Then drip a bit of 3% hydrogen peroxide into one ear. After a few moments you will hear fizzing. Wait until the fizzing stops -- 10 to 15 minutes, occasionally adding more hydrogen peroxide. Shake remaining liquid from your ear onto the towel and repeat on the other ear.

Eczema

Eczema, with its itchy skin, is a fairly common condition especially in children, but can become severe with skin becoming broken, raw, and bleeding.

BEST REMEDIES:

- **Apple Cider Vinegar:** Drinking and applying apple cider vinegar (ACV) can restore your overall skin health and stop eczema rashes. Dilute a bit of ACV 1:1 with water and wash eczema patches with it, while also taking a daily ACV tonic—one teaspoon of ACV in a large glass of water (natural sweetener to taste, optional). Increase the amount of ACV to 1-2 tablespoons per glass as your body tolerates it.
- **Coconut Oil:** Apply natural coconut oil directly on your eczema patches just as you would a lotion. It's an excellent all-around skin care product! You can also add up to a tablespoon of coconut oil to your daily diet for better skin and general health.

Exercise-Induced Urticaria

Hives can at times be brought on by vigorous exercise (Exercise-Induced Urticaria), resulting in raised patches of red skin that can appear anywhere on the body. Such hives are often very itchy.

BEST REMEDY:

- **Apple Cider Vinegar:** Drinking and applying apple cider vinegar (ACV) can restore your overall skin health and stop the hives. Dilute a bit of ACV 1:1 with water and wash patches of hives with it to stop the itch and help in healing. Also consider taking a daily ACV tonic—one teaspoon of ACV in a large glass of water (natural sweetener to taste, optional). Increase the amount of ACV to 1-2 tablespoons per glass as your body tolerates it.

Eyes, Dry

Dry eyes are increasingly common, with so many of us sitting in front of computers all day. It can be a congenital condition that results in reduced tear production, or may just be an environmental effect. In either case, the irritation and redness can be uncomfortable and eventually damage the eye.

BEST REMEDY:
- **Fish Oil:** Taking fish oil pills (as directed) can help your body's own self-lubricating systems take care of your eyes and end the dry eye symptoms.

Eyes, Infections

Conjunctivitis is better known as 'pink eye', and is a viral infection that causes irritation, watering, reddening of the eyes, and a distinct pinkness to the eye's conjunctiva (the combined area at the edge of the eye and on the inside of the eyelid). A bacterial form is also possible.

BEST REMEDIES:
- **Apple Cider Vinegar:** Mix about two teaspoons of unpasteurized apple cider vinegar in a cup of water, then dip a cotton pad or soft cloth in it to wash the eyelid inside and out. You can place a few drops of the water mixture in the eye as well. Repeat every few hours until the conjunctivitis is all gone, usually 2-3 days.
- **Green Tea Bags:** Put two green tea bags in a cup of hot water and allow the tea to brew and then cool somewhat,

then apply each bag to an eye. Rewarm in the water and continue for about 10 minutes. Repeat every few hours until healed, usually 2-3 days.

- **Colloidal Silver:** Place a drop of colloidal silver in the affected eye 2-3 times a day until symptoms are gone.
- **Sea Salt:** Combine a tablespoon of sea salt in a cup of water and apply 2-3 drops to the corners of your eyes first thing in the morning and last thing at night.
- **Black Tea Bag:** Make a cup of black tea and allow it to cool a bit. Then apply the tea bag to the eye and keep it there for ten minutes or so. Repeat every few hours for the 1-3 days it will take to clear up the conjunctivitis.

Fatigue

Chronic fatigue is an increasingly common symptom, sometimes seen in sufferers of fibromyalgia, adrenal fatigue, and other conditions.

BEST REMEDY:

- **Apple Cider Vinegar and Baking Soda:** One-quarter teaspoon of baking soda with up to two tablespoons of apple cider vinegar (ACV) in a large glass of water can be an excellent overall health tonic, addressing the multiple causes that lead to chronic fatigue. Try starting with just one teaspoon of ACV, then working your way up (and watch out for the fizz!).

Fever

The body uses fever to fight infections and prevent bacteria or viruses from overtaking the body. However, when a fever gets too high or lasts too long it can weaken the body and even cause direct damage to the brain and other organs.

BEST REMEDIES:

- **Egg Whites:** By far the most popular natural fever remedy! To quickly reduce a fever, soak a paper towel in egg whites and apply the paper to the feet. Keep the paper wet with new egg whites as needed until the fever breaks.
- **Potato:** Cut two thick, long slices out of a potato, place them on the soles of the feet, and then slide socks overtop both foot and potato. Leave them there until the fever subsides, often very quickly. For added effectiveness, place the slices in the refrigerator for a while first!
- **Apple Cider Vinegar:** Apple cider vinegar can quickly reduce a fever. Either add a cup to a warm bath or soak

two washcloths in the vinegar—one to lay on the forehead and one on the stomach.

Fibroid Tumors

While uterine fibroids are common, benign tumors (affecting 25-50% of women) they can cause secondary conditions and worsen the symptoms of a period.

BEST REMEDIES:
- **Blackstrap Molasses:** Adding a tablespoon of blackstrap molasses (not the typical stuff you find in the grocery store) to your daily diet can give your body the rich source of nutrients and minerals (iron aplenty) that your body needs. Many people like it in coffee or milk and find that their symptoms and perhaps the fibroids themselves decrease drastically.
- **Apple Cider Vinegar:** A daily apple cider vinegar (ACV) tonic can reduce fibroid symptoms and perhaps the tumors themselves. Mix one teaspoon of ACV in a large glass of water (natural sweetener to taste, optional) and drink. Increase the amount of ACV to 1-2 tablespoons per glass as your body tolerates it.

Fibrocystic Breast Disease

Many women experience a monthly change in the breast tissue where fibrous lumps form in the area of the breasts nearest the armpits. While they are non-cancerous and do not interfere with breast-feeding, they and the nipples can be itchy and tender with a feeling of fullness in the breasts.

BEST REMEDY:
- **Iodine:** Iodine pills or Lugol's iodine drops can be taken as directed to reduce or eliminate the fibrocystic symptoms (kelp tablets are also an option).

Flu

Influenza, the common flu, is an annual threat to worldwide health, especially among the youngest and oldest among us. Accompanied by fever and aching as well as the typical cold symptoms, the flu can progress to become pneumonia, a far more serious condition.

BEST REMEDIES:
- **Apple Cider Vinegar:** Take a tablespoon each of apple cider vinegar and honey in a warm but not hot glass of water up to three times a day to relieve all flu symptoms, including sore throat.
- **Hydrogen Peroxide:** At the first sign of the flu, lie on your side and put a few drops of 3% hydrogen peroxide in your ear, and then let it sit for several minutes. Then empty out that ear and repeat on the other side. Hydrogen peroxide's antiviral properties seem to cut the flu virus down before it can take hold.
- **Grapefruit Seed Extract:** A few drops of grapefruit seed extract, taken as directed, can stop a flu in its tracks and greatly reduce flu symptoms.
- **Hydrogen Peroxide Inhalation:** While it should be undertaken carefully, using an emptied, boiling water sterilized nasal spray bottle to inhale 3% hydrogen peroxide can open up airways and reduce flu symptoms. (Be sure to first sterilize the spray bottle with boiling water.) Point the spray bottle in your mouth and at the back of your throat, and while inhaling sharply pump 4-6 sprays of the hydrogen peroxide. Repeat 4-6 times a day.

Fluid Retention

Bloating and fluid retention can be uncomfortable and make it tough to get into our favorite clothes! It's usually a sign of some imbalance in the body.

BEST REMEDY:
- **Apple Cider Vinegar:** A daily ACV tonic can restore your body's mineral balance and reduce bloating. Start with one teaspoon of apple cider vinegar in a tall glass of water and build up to as much as two tablespoons. Take a few days off the tonic every so often.

Folliculitis

Folliculitis is an infection of the hair follicles, usually caused by bacteria. Folliculitis commonly looks like red pimples with a hair in the center of each one. These pimples may have pus in them and they often itch or burn. Besides bacteria, the condition can also be caused by a fungus or yeast.

BEST REMEDY:
- **Turmeric:** Adding one teaspoon of turmeric to your daily diet can cure and prevent folliculitis. While it is good in many foods, you can also add the teaspoonful to a glass of milk or water. Also available in pill form.

Food Poisoning

Everyone has been laid low by food poisoning at one time or another. Leading to diarrhea and vomiting in most cases, it can at times result in death.

BEST REMEDIES:
- **Apple Cider Vinegar:** Immediately taking 2 tablespoons of apple cider vinegar (straight, ideally, in a glass of water if you must) can kill off foreign pathogens in your food and stop food poisoning in no time at all.
- **Activated Charcoal:** The incredible absorbency of activated charcoal powder can suck up the pathogens that cause food poisoning and bring swift relief. Activated charcoal capsules are available at the drug store.

Fungus, Nails

Yellowed, thickened nails are the most obvious sign of a fungus infection around your finger or toenails. A small white or yellow spot underneath a nail may be the first sign of fungal infection.

BEST REMEDIES:

- **Apple Cider Vinegar:** A daily apple cider vinegar (ACV) tonic (up to two tablespoons of ACV in a tall glass of water) and daily ACV soak of the affected nails (mix water and ACV 2:1 in a basin and soak for 10-20 minutes) can kill nail fungus. Be aware that the ACV soak can further discolor the nails.
- **Oil of Oregano:** Used as directed internally and externally, oil of oregano can be a very effective anti-fungal, although it is a bit expensive. Mix with a kitchen oil to apply to the affected nail.
- **Lemongrass Essential Oil:** Lemongrass essential oil can be mixed with a kitchen oil (mix about 12 drops to an ounce of oil) and applied directly to the affected nail twice a day to kill off a fungal infection. You will need to reapply for several weeks until the infection is completely gone.
- **Hydrogen Peroxide:** Use a cotton swab to apply 3% hydrogen peroxide directly to the affected nail (not the skin!) twice a day to kill nail fungus within a couple of weeks.
- **Tea Tree Oil:** Use a cotton swab to apply tea tree oil directly to the affected nail 2-3 times a day for several weeks until the fungus is completely eradicated.
- **Distilled Vinegar:** Cheaper than apple cider vinegar, regular distilled vinegar works for many people to kill off a nail fungus infection. Simply mix water and white vinegar in a 2:1 solution (mostly water) and soak the affected nails for 10-20 minutes once or twice daily until the infection clears. You can also dab vinegar directly on the infected nails.

- **Mouthwash:** Soak a cotton ball in an alcohol-based mouthwash and hold the cotton to the affected nail for at least 10-20 minutes once or twice a day. In 2-3 weeks, the infection should be eliminated and the nails on their way to recovery.
- **Iodine:** Apply iodine to the fungus-infected nails and the skin around them once a day as an antifungal agent. Within a few weeks, the infection should be gone. Colorless iodine is available.

G

Gall Bladder Attacks

The growth of gallstones in the gallbladder can result in gallbladder attacks, painful episodes that often follow fatty meals. It can be accompanied by nausea and vomiting.

BEST REMEDY:
- **Apple Cider Vinegar in Apple Juice:** To stop a gallstone attack, add 1-3 tablespoons of unpasteurized apple cider vinegar to a glass of apple juice and drink. Relief should come quickly!

Gallstones

Gallstones can accumulate and grow in the gallbladder for some time before they become symptomatic. Once they do, the intense and lasting pain (often following a fatty meal) can be impossible to ignore. Nausea and vomiting are also possible.

BEST REMEDY:
- **Gallbladder Cleanses:** For long-term relief from gall bladder attacks, Hulda Clark's olive oil and lemon juice liver and gall bladder cleanse seems to be the most effective option. However, it is a somewhat complicated remedy, so please find a reputable online source for the cleanse and follow it closely.

Gas / Flatulence

Gas, or flatulence, is a normal byproduct of digestion. However, substantial amounts or particularly odorous gas can be embarrassing, uncomfortable, and inconvenient. It may also be a symptom of a larger digestive issue.

BEST REMEDY:
- **Apple Cider Vinegar:** Adding the apple cider vinegar (ACV) tonic to your daily diet can increase your digestive acids and enzymes, help cleanse your digestive track, and thereby reduce the amount of gas your body produces. Take one teaspoon of ACV (natural sweetener optional) and mix it in a large glass of water. Drink with breakfast or each meal of the day. Increase the ACV in each glass to as much as 2 tablespoons.

Genital Warts

The highly contagious HPV virus can cause genital warts in the exposed person. Very small warts or larger clusters can form throughout the genital and anal area, and they can spread HPV to sexual partners through skin-to-skin contact.

BEST REMEDIES:
- **Apple Cider Vinegar:** An exceedingly popular remedy, apple cider vinegar (ACV) can be very effective within a few days. Simply soak a cotton ball in ACV and apply to the warts. You can use a band-aid to hold the cotton to the wart for a few hours at a time. Okay for internal use, though there will be significant discomfort at first.
- **Garlic:** Scrape the skin off one edge of a clove of garlic and apply it directly to the genital wart. It will burn, but you can leave it on the wart for perhaps an hour at a time, reapplying several times throughout the day.

Genital Herpes

Caused by Herpes simplex virus (HSV) 2, genital herpes is characterized by clusters of inflamed skin that look like cold sores. The sufferer may also experience itching, burning, and pain whenever the recurring infection acts up.

BEST REMEDIES:

- **Apple Cider Vinegar:** Use a cotton swab to apply apple cider vinegar to any lesions 3-4 times a day. There will be a bit of a burn, but the herpes outbreak should clear in 2-3 days.
- **Bach Flower Remedies:** Commercially available, the all-natural Bach Flower Remedies are flower extracts (those with the greatest potency are provided by Healing Herbs of Hereford, England). When used to heal cold sores and herpes, you should take the remedies both internally and externally. The most potent flower remedies to heal herpes are holly, walnut, and crab apple. Any one of the three will work by itself. You can also take the three together in a formula.
- **L-Lysine:** You can take the essential amino acid L-Lysine in tablet form daily as directed to quickly heal a herpes outbreak and prevent further outbreaks from occurring with regular use. Try 1000mg daily for regular use and hourly during an outbreak, then adjust to your body's needs.
- **Coconut Oil:** Apply coconut oil directly to herpes sores 2-3 times a day, like a lotion. It works fast! You can also add a tablespoon of coconut oil to your daily diet to prevent future outbreaks.
- **Hydrogen Peroxide:** Use a cotton swab to apply 3% hydrogen peroxide directly to genital herpes sores to soothe the itch and pain. Do it 3-4 times a day or more and you should see significant reduction within a day or two.
- **Prunella Vulgaris:** Prunella vulgaris is the Latin name for a medicinal plant otherwise known as Heal-All. You can get it in supplement form and take it daily as directed.

Gout

Gout is an arthritis-like condition where a buildup of crystals of uric acid in the body causes pain, swelling, stiffness, and other symptoms in certain joints of the body.

BEST REMEDIES:

- **Apple Cider Vinegar:** Taking an apple cider vinegar (ACV) tonic 1-3 times daily can improve your overall nutrition and help dissolve the uric acid crystals. Mix a teaspoon of ACV in a large glass of water (honey optional) and drink with a meal. Increase the amount of ACV as high as 2 tablespoons per glass, as your body requires.
- **Cherries:** A classic home remedy, eating tart cherries (low in sugar) can relieve a gout attack within a couple of days. Tart cherry extract in pill form is also available to prevent gout over the long term.
- **Black Bean Broth:** Make a batch of simple black bean soup and then separate out the dark broth. Drinking this broth can quickly dissolve crystalline uric acid, thanks to the anthocyanins contained in the skins of the black beans.

Grey Hair

Grey hair is not inevitable, and at the very least it can be delayed if the "root" cause is a vitamin or other dietary deficiency, which is often the case.

BEST REMEDY:

- **Blackstrap Molasses:** Nutrient and mineral rich blackstrap molasses undergoes an additional refining step over the stuff you ordinarily find in the grocery store. Adding a daily tablespoon of blackstrap molasses to your diet can restore needed nutrients to your body, slowing and perhaps reversing your hair's transition to grey. Many people like the taste of it in coffee!

Gum Disease

Gum disease, or gingivitis, is the inflammation of the gums due to plaque. The plaques release toxins that irritate and degrade the gums and teeth.

BEST REMEDIES:

- **Hydrogen Peroxide:** Mix 3% hydrogen peroxide in a 1:1 solution with water and use as an occasional mouthwash. The hydrogen peroxide will kill the damaging bacteria that cause plaque and infect the gums.
- **Oil Pulling:** The ancient practice of oil pulling is finding renewed fame for its ability to pull toxins out of the body. Before brushing your teeth and with an empty stomach, take one Tbsp of oil into your mouth and swish it around for 10-20 minutes until the oil has turned milky white. Then spit out. Most any food oil can do, but sesame and sunflower oils are traditional and the most popular.
- **Turmeric:** Gum disease, especially bleeding along the gumline, can be addressed by applying a bit of turmeric powder to a toothbrush and brushing as usual. You can use daily, but turmeric will stain your toothbrush yellow. You should also continue brushing with regular toothpaste as well.

Hair Loss

Hair Thinning, Baldness, Male Pattern Baldness & Hair Loss are all fairly common but not inevitable. Hair loss is sometimes genetic, but also caused by illness, malnutrition, nutrient deficiencies, stress, and other causes.

BEST REMEDIES:
- **Apple Cider Vinegar:** Adding the apple cider vinegar (ACV) tonic to your daily diet can increase your digestive acids and enzymes, improving your overall nutrition and health thereby giving your body the ability to grow a healthy head of hair. Take one teaspoon of ACV (honey optional) and mix it in a large glass of water. Drink with breakfast or each meal of the day. Increase the ACV in each glass to as much as 2 tablespoons.
- **Coconut Oil:** Add up to one tablespoon of coconut oil to your daily diet to improve your nutrition and give your scalp the raw materials it needs to prevent hair loss. You can also rub coconut oil into your scalp as a lotion for your skin and hair alike. Very effective!

Halitosis

Bad breath, formally known as halitosis, can come from a variety of causes including digestion issues. However, an oral source of bad breath is reasonably common.

BEST REMEDY:
- **Hydrogen Peroxide:** A mouthwash made of 3% hydrogen peroxide and water in a 1:1 solution can be used occasionally to kill off the offensive bacteria that are causing your bad breath.

Hayfever

Hay fever and seasonal allergies can be an annual nightmare for some of us, but a few natural remedies can prevent allergy attacks or at least reduce allergic symptoms.

BEST REMEDIES:
- **Apple Cider Vinegar:** A bit of apple cider vinegar in a tall glass of water once a day can stop an allergy attack and reduce seasonal allergy symptoms. Start with one teaspoon and built up to as much as two tablespoons. You can add a touch of raw local honey as well for added effect.
- **Turmeric:** It's not exactly a spoonful of sugar, but a teaspoon of turmeric powder in a glass of water can stop a dripping nose and sore throat due to allergies. Turmeric in capsule form is also available from health food stores.
- **Honey:** Enjoying some raw local honey (or chewing honeycomb) before the start of allergy season can give your body a sort of vaccination to prevent or reduce seasonal allergy symptoms. Try one teaspoon at bedtime to combat allergies and help you sleep better as well!

Headaches

Head pain is an extremely common complaint but one that can be incredibly disruptive. Stress, diet, eye strain, dehydration, and sinus issues are common causes.

BEST REMEDIES:
- **Apple Cider Vinegar:** At the onset of a headache, take a tablespoon each of apple cider vinegar and honey mixed in a large glass of water. This should prevent a headache, and it can be taken 1-3 times a day as needed.
- **Cayenne Pepper:** Snorting a quarter teaspoon of powdered cayenne pepper up the nose can cure a headache in minutes, especially if it is a sinus headache or related condition.

- **Acupressure:** Hitting the right acupressure points can relieve headache pain quickly and lastingly. Try pinching the area between your thumb and forefinger for five minutes. Or hold one thumb against your head directly between the eyes and the other at the base of your skull, just where the spine enters, and count to ten before releasing.

Heartburn

Digestion issues can cause your stomach to release stomach acids up the esophagus, resulting in heartburn—a burning pain behind the sternum, sometimes rising up the throat and jaw.

BEST REMEDIES:
- **Apple Cider Vinegar:** To stop an attack of heartburn, take a tall glass of water and add one tablespoon each of honey and apple cider vinegar. Drinking this ACV tonic can bring heartburn relief. Taken with meals, it can stop heartburn before it starts.
- **Mustard:** To stop a case of heartburn, swallow 1-4 teaspoons of yellow mustard. It will get worse before it gets better, but relief will quickly follow!

Heart Palpitations

Ordinarily, we pay little attention to the beating of our own hearts. A palpitation is any time that we do suddenly become aware of that heartbeat, whether it be too fast, too slow, irregular, a missed beat, or even at its normal pace.

BEST REMEDIES:
- **Blackstrap Molasses:** Blackstrap molasses (more concentrated than most grocery store offerings) is rich in iron, magnesium, and other nutrients that can help in proper heart functioning. Add a tablespoon of molasses to your daily diet for continued heart health.

- **Magnesium:** Taking magnesium supplements or using Transdermal Magnesium Therapy to restore necessary magnesium reserves can quiet heart palpitations. Magnesium is a critical component of proper muscle functioning.

Heel Spurs

Heel spurs, calcified growths on the heel bone, are often accompanied by plantar fasciitis, a painful inflammation of the connective tissue supporting the arch of your foot. Most often, the pain is felt directly beneath the heel.

BEST REMEDY:
- **Apple Cider Vinegar Wrap:** Soak a cloth or bandage in apple cider vinegar and apply to the heel. You can leave it on for several hours, even wrap a plastic bag around heel and cloth to sleep with it at night. The pain should recede quickly and the underlying condition should be gone within a few weeks of daily treatment.

Hemorrhoids

Hemorrhoids are an inflammation of the veins around the rectum and anus, resulting in itching and discomfort. It is a condition that can become severe and require surgery.

BEST REMEDIES:
- **Apple Cider Vinegar:** Soak cotton or toilet paper in apple cider vinegar (ACV) and apply it to the hemorrhoid, leaving it there for as long as practicable. The pain and itch should be relieved almost on contact, and after a few applications the inflammation should go away. You can also add half a cup of ACV to a sitz bath.
- **Rutin:** Rutin is a natural component of many plants, including buckwheat, cranberries, and asparagus. It has a number of proven, positive effects on the health of the

circulatory system. You can get it in pill form and use as directed to treat hemorrhoids.

- **Castor Oil:** As a variation of a castor oil pack, take a square of toilet paper and soak it in castor oil. Apply the soaked paper on the hemorrhoids and leave in place until your next trip to the bathroom. Relief is often immediate, but you can reapply if need be.
- **Coconut Oil:** Apply coconut oil directly to hemorrhoids like a lotion and reapply whenever convenient to quickly soothe the itching and pain. The hemorrhoids themselves should vanish within several days.

Herpes (oral)

Cold sores, caused by the herpes simplex virus, are fairly common but nonetheless irritating and embarrassing. We have found that they are triggered and exacerbated by artificial sweeteners. Yet one more reason to avoid them!

BEST REMEDIES:
- **Acetone Nail Polish Remover:** Use a cotton swab to apply a bit of acetone nail polish remover to a cold sore about once an hour until the cold sore is gone—often in a day or two!
- **Hydrogen Peroxide:** Dip a cotton swab in hydrogen peroxide and apply to any cold sore every few hours throughout the day to get rid of a cold sore within about three days.
- **Apple Cider Vinegar:** You'll feel a bit of a burning at first, but if you dab a bit of apple cider vinegar on a cold sore, it should dry out and disappear within about three days. Reapply about 4-5 times a day.
- **Ear Wax:** Odd but true! As soon as you get a cold sore tingle, apply a bit of your own earwax to the spot to stop the eruption from ever forming. Works even after the cold sore has formed. Leave it on, but don't lick your lips (yuck!).

- **L-Lysine:** Start taking the essential amino acid L-Lysine (in pill form) as soon as you feel a cold sore forming. You can reduce the number/size of cold stores or stop the outbreak entirely.
- **Garlic:** Cut a clove of garlic in small pieces and hold a piece to your cold sore for about ten minutes, 3-5 times a day (no more!) to dry out your cold sore and kill the virus at the same time.
- **Coconut Oil:** Adding up to a tablespoonful of cold pressed coconut oil to your daily diet (start with an eighth of a teaspoonful and increase slowly) can put an end to your cold sore attacks. For an active cold sore, try applying coconut oil directly to the sore a few times a day and leaving there.

Herpes (genital)

Caused by Herpes simplex virus (HSV) 2, genital herpes is characterized by clusters of inflamed skin that look like cold sores. The sufferer may also experience itching, burning, and pain whenever the recurring infection acts up.

BEST REMEDIES:

- **Apple Cider Vinegar:** Use a cotton swab to apply apple cider vinegar to any lesions 3-4 times a day. There will be a bit of a burn, but the herpes outbreak should clear in 2-3 days.
- **Bach Flower Remedies:** Commercially available, the all-natural Bach Flower Remedies are flower extracts (the most potent extracts are available from Healing Herbs of Hereford, England). When used to heal cold sores and herpes, you should take the remedies both internally and externally. The most potent flower remedies to heal herpes are holly, walnut, and crab apple. Any one of the three will work by itself. You can also take the three together in a formula.

- **L-Lysine:** You can take the essential amino acid L-Lysine in tablet form daily as directed to quickly heal a herpes outbreak and prevent further outbreaks from occurring with regular use. Try 1000mg daily for regular use and hourly during an outbreak, then adjust to your body's needs.
- **Coconut Oil:** Apply coconut oil directly to herpes sores 2-3 times a day, like a lotion. It works fast! You can also add a tablespoon of coconut oil to your daily diet to prevent future outbreaks.
- **Hydrogen Peroxide:** Use a cotton swab to apply 3% hydrogen peroxide directly to genital herpes sores to soothe the itch and pain. Do it 3-4 times a day or more and you should see significant reduction within a day or two.
- **Prunella Vulgaris:** Prunella vulgaris is the Latin name for a medicinal plant otherwise known as Heal-All. You can get it in supplement form and take it daily as directed.

Hiccups

Everyone knows a few traditional remedies to cure the hiccups, but which ones actually work? According to our online community, these are the best hiccup cures.

BEST REMEDIES:
- **Holding the Breath:** Take in three large breaths, then hold the last breath for as long as possible. Repeat if necessary.
- **Drink Upside Down:** Get a bit of water in your mouth, bend over so that the top of your head is pointed at the ground, and then swallow while still upside down.
- **Vinegar:** Drink a teaspoon of vinegar to instantly cure hiccups. According to some, it can be mixed with sugar to dull the taste!
- **Sugar:** Swallow a teaspoon of sugar all at once to quickly cure hiccups.
- **Peanut Butter:** Eat a tablespoonful of peanut butter in one mouthful to reset the diaphragm and cure hiccups.

Hidradenitis Suppurativa

In some people, the sweat glands and some hair follicles can become clogged and swollen with pus. These cysts eventually burst and drain. This can occur in the armpits, groin and thighs, or beneath the breasts and can result in scarring.

BEST REMEDY:
- **Turmeric:** Turmeric capsules are available, but you can also simply take 1 tsp of powdered turmeric in 1/4 cup of water three times day. Many people also like it in warm milk (almond or rice will do as well as dairy).

High Blood Pressure

High blood pressure (above 120/80), known as hypertension, is a critical health concern that can lead to heart conditions, stroke, and other significant health concerns.

BEST REMEDIES:
- **Apple Cider Vinegar:** Taking the ACV tonic 2-3 times a day can significantly lower your blood pressure. Start with one teaspoon of apple cider vinegar in a large glass of water and build up to one or two tablespoons. Add honey or other natural sweetener for taste.
- **Cayenne Pepper:** Cayenne pepper pills are available, but simply adding a teaspoon of cayenne to one of your daily meals can significantly reduce blood pressure almost immediately. Try adding it to hot water for an invigorating beverage!
- **Garlic:** A clove of raw garlic each day (or garlic tablets) can lower blood pressure effectively. Try a bit of fennel or parsley to block the garlic breath afterwards!
- **Apple Cider Vinegar and Baking Soda:** Add an eighth of a teaspoon of baking soda to the standard ACV tonic (two teaspoons of apple cider vinegar in a large glass of water) for a blood pressure remedy that is even more effective for some people than the straight tonic.

High Cholesterol

Cholesterol is simply a type of fat (a lipid) found in many foods. High cholesterol levels in the body and bloodstream, however, can result in clogged arteries (atherosclerosis), contributing to heart disease and the possibility of a heart attack or stroke.

BEST REMEDIES:

- **Apple Cider Vinegar:** To lower your overall cholesterol levels in short time, take the Apple Cider Vinegar tonic 2-3 times daily with meals. Start with one teaspoon apple cider vinegar in a tall glass of water (natural sweetener optional), and slowly increase the amount of vinegar to as much as 2 tablespoons per glass according to your body's needs.
- **Red Yeast Rice:** Red yeast rice is the newest discovery in natural cholesterol treatment. Available in tablets, take as directed.
- **Coconut Oil:** It may seem counterintuitive to add an oil to your diet to lower cholesterol, but many have been able to lower their LDLs with just the addition of Extra Virgin Coconut Oil to their diet. Start with ¼ teaspoon a day and slowly increase to as much as a daily tablespoon.

Hives

Hives are ordinarily the result of an allergic reaction. They are characterized by raised red skin that can be itchy, sting, or burn.

BEST REMEDY:

- **Apple Cider Vinegar:** Drinking and applying apple cider vinegar (ACV) can restore your overall skin health and stop the hives. Dilute a bit of ACV 1:1 with water and wash patches of hives with it to stop the itch and help in healing. Also consider taking a daily ACV tonic—one teaspoon of ACV in a large glass of water (natural sweetener to taste, optional). Increase the amount of ACV to 1-2 tablespoons per glass as your body tolerates it.

HPV with Genital Warts

The highly contagious HPV virus can cause genital warts in the exposed person. Very small warts or larger clusters can form throughout the genital and anal area, and they can spread HPV to sexual partners through skin-to-skin contact.

BEST REMEDIES:

- **Apple Cider Vinegar:** An exceedingly popular remedy, apple cider vinegar (ACV) can be very effective within a few days. Simply soak a cotton ball in ACV and apply to the warts. You can use a band-aid to hold the cotton to the wart for a few hours at a time. Okay for internal use, though there will be significant discomfort at first.
- **Garlic:** Scrape the skin off one edge of a clove of garlic and apply it directly to the genital wart. It will burn, but you can leave it on the wart for perhaps an hour at a time, reapplying several times throughout the day.

Hot Flashes

The hormonal changes that accompany menopause often result in hot flashes, a symptom in which the person suddenly becomes intensely hot, sweats, and experiences a rising heart rate. This may last for up to half an hour and recur several times throughout the day.

BEST REMEDY:

- **Apple Cider Vinegar:** To steady your metabolism and reduce or eliminate hot flashes, mix 2 teaspoons of apple cider vinegar in 16 ounces of water that you'll sip throughout the day. You will be keeping your pH in a constant, alkalized state by sipping this highly diluted dosage. Usually 1-2 tall glasses of the concoction are all you'll need each day.

Hypothyroidism

Hypothyroidism, a lack of certain hormones due to a low-functioning thyroid gland, can be the result of a number of conditions. It can have a number of early symptoms including fatigue, cold intolerance, constipation, thin and brittle fingernails, paleness, itchy skin, and weight gain.

BEST REMEDY:
- **Coconut Oil:** Add up to a tablespoon of coconut oil to your daily diet to get the general health benefits of this remarkable dietary aid and to improve thyroid function.

IBS

Irritable Bowel Syndrome (IBS) seems to be increasingly common. Sufferers may experience bloating, changes in bowel habits, and pain on defecation.

BEST REMEDY:

- **Apple Cider Vinegar:** The mix of nutrients and digestive aids in unpasteurized apple cider vinegar (ACV) can slow the digestive process, improve intestinal metabolism, and regulate the excretory system. Take the ACV tonic three times a day with meals—one teaspoon of ACV in a large glass of water (honey optional). Increase the amount of ACV to 1-2 tablespoons per glass as your body tolerates it.

Infertility

A man or woman's inability to create children can be the result of any number of biological causes. Addressing an existing imbalance or nutritional deficiency may help.

BEST REMEDY:

- **Apple Cider Vinegar:** The body's pH balance is a critical thing, and an imbalance in pH levels in any part of the body could be a barrier to pregnancy. Drinking a daily ACV (apple cider vinegar) tonic can help restore pH balance. Mix 2 teaspoons of apple cider vinegar in 16 ounces of water that you'll sip throughout the day. You will be keeping your pH in a constant, alkalized state by sipping this highly diluted dosage. Usually 1-2 tall glasses of the concoction are all you'll need each day.

Insomnia

The inability to fall asleep or stay asleep, no matter the cause, is called insomnia. Pain is the most frequent cause but medications, stress, and environmental changes are among the very many other causes.

BEST REMEDIES:
- **Apple Cider Vinegar:** Restoring your body's pH and nutritive balance might be all you need for a good night's sleep. Try adding an apple cider vinegar (ACV) tonic to your daily routine—Mix 2 teaspoons of apple cider vinegar in 16 ounces of water that you'll sip throughout the day. You will be keeping your pH in a constant, alkalized state by sipping this highly diluted dosage. Usually 1-2 tall glasses of the concoction are all you'll need each day.
- **Ear Plugs:** Blocking out the distracting sounds of the world can be the easiest way to get some much needed sleep.
- **Melatonin:** Melatonin tablets, taken as directed, are a popular natural remedy for sleeplessness. It is a hormone that naturally occurs in the human body, helping to regulate the circadian (and thus sleep) rhythms.

Itchy Skin

Dry and itchy skin is about as common a condition as you can get, though drier climates and colder winter seasons can exacerbate the problem. Too much sun exposure, change in diet, medications, and any number of other influences can cause temporary itching as well.

BEST REMEDY:
- **Apple Cider Vinegar:** Soak a cloth in apple cider vinegar and place it on the itchy skin for 15 minutes or more to soothe itchy skin. The vinegar's nutrients and antibiotic potency can potentially remedy the underlying cause, in addition.

J

Joint Pain

Arthritis is not the only cause of joint pain. Gout, bursitis, degenerative bone conditions, injury, infection, and illnesses are also possible causes.

BEST REMEDIES:

- **Apple Cider Vinegar:** A daily apple cider vinegar (ACV) tonic can target joint pain in a number of ways—by dissolving joint deposits, improving lubricants, reducing swelling, and generally by aiding in nutrition. Mix 2 teaspoons of apple cider vinegar in 16 ounces of water that you'll sip throughout the day. You will be keeping your pH in a constant, alkalized state by sipping this highly diluted dosage. Usually 1-2 tall glasses of the concoction are all you'll need each day.

- **Turmeric:** Turmeric is a powerful antioxidant and general health aid. Add one teaspoonful each of turmeric powder and honey to a warm glass of milk (almond or rice will do as well as dairy) for daily use. Also available in pill form.

K

Keratosis Pilaris

Keratosis pilaris, commonly known as "chicken skin", is harmless but can be found unattractive. It consists of raised bumps around the hair follicles on the backs of the arms, thighs, and sometimes other parts of the body.

BEST REMEDY:
- **Apple Cider Vinegar:** Apply apple cider vinegar to the affected skin just like a body wash and then either leave on or rinse off. Many report having smooth skin within days.

Kidney Stones

Minerals dissolved in the urine can solidify and build into stones within the kidneys. These can eventually be passed, though if they become sufficiently large that passage can block the urethra and cause significant pain.

BEST REMEDIES:
- **Olive Oil and Lemon Juice:** Exceedingly popular remedy! Mix two ounces each of freshly squeezed lemon juice and olive oil. Drink this (not nearly as bad as you think) and follow it up with plenty of water. You can repeat this 2-3 times a day until the stones pass, which often happens within 1-3 days.
- **Apple Cider Vinegar:** To dissolve and pass a kidney stone with limited discomfort, mix 2 oz. of apple cider vinegar in a glass of water and drink over a short period of time. Repeat the next day if necessary, but this will often help you to pass kidney stones within a day's time.
- **Lemons:** Mix at least 4 oz. of lemon juice in a glass of water and drink once a day until the acidic lemon juice

helps to break up the kidney stones and allows them to pass.

- **Chanca Piedra:** Chanca piedra, a plant whose name actually means stone breaker, is an effective natural remedy for kidney stones. Find the pills at a local health store or online and take as directed.

Knees - Bad or Weak

Knees are complicated joints with many moving parts that can get out of whack, resulting in pain and weakness that can sometimes be remedied by changes or additions to your diet.

BEST REMEDIES:
- **Apple Cider Vinegar:** Mix 2 teaspoons of apple cider vinegar in 16 ounces of water that you'll sip throughout the day. You will be keeping your pH in a constant, alkalized state by sipping this highly diluted dosage. Usually 1-2 tall glasses of the concoction are all you'll need each day. This can help dissolve mineral build-ups within the joint and help restore joint lubricants.
- **Omega 3 Supplements:** Fish oil or flaxseed oil will provide your body with needed omega 3 fatty acids. Along with a host of other benefits, these omega 3's can restore some of the cushioning components of the joints. Just be careful that you get pharmaceutical grade fish oil if you choose fish over flaxseed, so as to avoid mercury and other heavy metal contaminants.
- **Weight Loss:** Losing just a few extra pounds can really take the pressure off your knees and reduce the impact of all that daily pounding and standing-around pressure on the joint.

L

Laryngitis

Any number of things can cause the inflammation of the larynx and irritation of the vocal cords that causes laryngitis—the inability to speak.

BEST REMEDY:
- **Apple Cider Vinegar and Cayenne:** Drink and gargle with the following mixture to soothe laryngitis and reduce inflammation—One tablespoon each of apple cider vinegar, powdered cayenne pepper, and honey mixed in a large glass of warm (not hot) water.

Lice

A case of lice can be itchy, irritating, and embarrassing. Head lice are insects that can be passed through shared clothing or close contact.

BEST REMEDY:
- **Mayonnaise:** Coat hair and scalp with ordinary mayonnaise and cover with plastic for a couple of hours. Then wash out. People report cures in a single application!

Low Energy

It can be frustrating not to have the energy to get through the day's normal activities, but a few changes to your diet might combat general or chronic fatigue.

BEST REMEDY:
- **Apple Cider Vinegar:** To boost your energy and keep it going all day, try Earth Clinic's most popular all around remedy. Mix 2 teaspoons of apple cider vinegar in 16

ounces of water that you'll sip throughout the day. You will be keeping your pH in a constant, alkalized state by sipping this highly diluted dosage. Usually 1-2 tall glasses of the concoction are all you'll need each day.

Lupus

Lupus is a chronic autoimmune disease where the body's immune system attacks itself. Most often affecting women, when lupus flares up it can inflame and do damage to any part of the body.

BEST REMEDIES:
- **Ted's Remedy:** Our resident natural remedies expert offers a regimen that has brought more relief to sufferers than any other Lupus remedy. Ted's remedy concentrates on a few supplements and aims to alkalize the body, since putting your body in an acidic state seems to worsen Lupus symptoms.
  - ◊ Twice daily, take a half-teaspoon of baking soda mixed in a small glass of water.
  - ◊ Vitamin D supplements. Take 2000 – 20,000 i.u./ day, especially during the winter.
  - ◊ Avoid B6 and nicotinic acid supplements, as they are acid forming.
  - ◊ Drink filtered water to reduce chlorine, fluoride, and heavy metals.
  - ◊ Reduce or eliminate acid-forming foods such as sweets, meats, oily foods, white flour, fried foods, etc.
  - ◊ Monitor your urine with pH strips to maintain a pH of 7.0 or greater through the above steps.

Lymph Nodes, Swollen

Swollen lymph nodes are a common indication of some infection or illness in the body, though the infection can also strike the lymphatic system itself.

BEST REMEDY:

- **Apple Cider Vinegar:** To reduce the swelling lymph nodes, try an ACV tonic—one tablespoon of apple cider vinegar (ACV) in a large glass of water (honey optional).

Melanoma

Melanoma is one type of skin cancer. It affects mostly exposed skin and more rarely the eyes and bowels. While it is a less common form of skin cancer, it causes the most skin cancer deaths, so before attempting an at-home remedy, check with your doctor to make certain that what you are looking at is benign. A malignant melanoma needs medical care, and even a benign skin cancer can become malignant.

BEST REMEDY:

- **Hydrogen Peroxide:** Soak a cotton swab in 3% hydrogen peroxide and "scratch" at the melanoma until it turns white in color (be careful to avoid normal tissue). Do this three times a day until the melanoma dries up and flakes off.

Menopause

The onset of menopause and its constant hormonal changes can cause significant symptoms that need to be addressed in order to enjoy a normal life. Counted among these issues are hot flashes, breast tenderness, irregular menstruation, vaginal dryness, osteoporosis, and heart disease.

BEST REMEDY:

- **Apple Cider Vinegar:** To address many menopause symptoms, including bleeding issues and hot flashes, try Earth Clinic's most popular all-around remedy. Mix 2 teaspoons of apple cider vinegar in 16 ounces of water that you'll sip throughout the day. You will be keeping your pH in a constant, alkalized state by sipping this highly diluted dosage. Usually 1-2 tall glasses of the concoction are all you'll need each day.

Menstruation Issues

While some cramping is normal for all women, dysmenorrhea, heavy bleeding, missed periods, extreme cramping, and other menstruation issues can make a woman's 'time of the month' unnecessarily challenging.

BEST REMEDIES:

- **Blackstrap Molasses:** Add 1 tsp to 1 Tbsp of blackstrap molasses (more concentrated than the kind you'll find on most grocery store shelves) to your daily diet. It's a strong taste, but you can combine it with many foods, and its rich mix of nutrients (and iron!) has brought many women dramatic relief.
- **Apple Cider Vinegar:** Many women have found quick relief from heavy bleeding, cramping, missed periods, and other menstruation concerns with the apple cider vinegar (ACV) tonic taken 1-3 times a day with meals. Mix 1 tsp - 2 Tbsp apple cider vinegar in a large glass of water, w/ or w/o honey, and sip slowly.

Menstrual Cramps

While some cramping is normal for all women, dysmenorrhea, heavy bleeding, missed periods, extreme cramping, and other menstruation issues can make a woman's 'time of the month' unnecessarily challenging.

BEST REMEDIES:

- **Blackstrap Molasses:** Add 1 tsp to 1 Tbsp of blackstrap molasses (more concentrated than the kind you'll find on most grocery store shelves) to your daily diet. It's a strong taste, but you can combine it with many foods, and its rich mix of nutrients (and iron!) has brought many women dramatic relief.
- **Apple Cider Vinegar:** Many women have found quick relief from heavy bleeding, cramping, missed periods, and other menstruation concerns with the apple cider vinegar

(ACV) tonic taken 1-3 times a day with meals. Mix 1 tsp - 2 Tbsp apple cider vinegar in a large glass of water, w/ or w/o honey, and sip slowly.

Migraines

While headache is the most common symptom of a migraine, it can also be accompanied by a visual aura, partial loss of vision, nausea and vomiting, sensitivities to light and sound, and other symptoms.

BEST REMEDY:

- **Apple Cider Vinegar:** To counteract an impending or existing migraine, mix one tablespoon each of apple cider vinegar and honey in a tall glass of water and drink. Can be taken daily to prevent recurring migraines, but for many people it is best only to take it when migraine symptoms first present themselves.

Moles

The small, dark spots on the skin that we call moles are the result of high concentrations of the pigment melanin. A mole is not a health concern unless it is in fact, or turns into, a melanoma. Any mole that is ragged on the edges, larger than a pencil eraser, or dramatically different from your other moles should be examined by a doctor.

BEST REMEDIES:

- **Apple Cider Vinegar:** Abrade the mole lightly with an emery board or the like, and then soak a cotton swab in apple cider vinegar. Avoiding the healthy skin, apply the vinegar to the mole until it turns white. You can do this several times a day, but take it slowly at first. The mole will scab over a bit and eventually begin to flake off, though you may still need to continue treatment until the mole is completely gone.
- **Garlic:** Abrade the mole lightly with an emery board or the like, then crush a clove of garlic. Use a cotton

swab to apply the garlic to the mole, being careful not to touch the healthy skin. You can use tape or a band-aid to hold the garlic in place, or simply reapply every few hours. The mole will scab over a bit and eventually begin to flake off, though you may still need to continue treatment until the mole is completely gone.

- **Iodine:** Apply a drop of iodine to your mole 2-3 times a day to soon remove the mole. Be careful of staining.
- **Bloodroot Paste:** Abrade the mole lightly with an emery board or the like, then crush a bit of bloodroot. Apply the bloodroot directly on the mole, being careful to avoid the healthy skin. Wash off after a reasonable bit of time and reapply several times a day. The mole will scab over a bit and eventually begin to flake off, though you may still need to continue treatment until the mole is completely gone.
- **Hydrogen Peroxide:** Abrade the mole lightly with an emery board or the like, then dip a cotton swab in 3% hydrogen peroxide. Apply directly to the mole, avoiding the healthy skin, and hold it there until the mole turns white. Repeat several times throughout the day. The mole will scab over a bit and eventually begin to flake off, though you may still need to continue treatment until the mole is completely gone.

Molluscum Contagiosum

Molluscum Contagiosum is a viral infection that appears fairly commonly in children and less often in adults. It is very infectious, but results only in solid-feeling bumps on the skin that generally are free of pain or irritation.

BEST REMEDY:
- **Apple Cider Vinegar:** Apply the antibacterial qualities of apple cider vinegar (ACV) to the task by soaking a cotton makeup swab in ACV and then taping it over the affected skin. You can leave it on overnight then reapply as

needed. The papules will turn white (possibly with black cores) and then fall off or disappear within several days.

Mononucleosis

Infectious mononucleosis (mono) is widely known as the "kissing disease" even though this label is only partly true. Kissing can indeed spread the virus (Epstein-Barr), but more commonly transmission occurs through coughing, sneezing, or sharing a cup.

BEST REMEDY:
- **Coconut Oil:** Consume 3-4 tablespoons of coconut oil daily while experiencing mono symptoms. You can take it straight, mixed as sweetener with hot tea, blended into a smoothie, etc. A powerful general health aid, coconut oil seems to have antiviral properties and more generally will banish the typical mononucleosis fatigue.

Mouth Ulcers

The painful oral ulcers of a canker sore outbreak can be isolated or coat the throat and mouth in open sores. While not contagious, the root cause of a canker sore is unknown.

BEST REMEDIES:
- **Apple Cider Vinegar:** For immediate relief, apply apple cider vinegar (ACV) directly to a canker sore. For long-term freedom from sores, try a daily ACV tonic—One teaspoon of ACV in a large glass of water. Increase the dose of ACV up to as much as two tablespoons, according to your body's needs.
- **Aspirin:** Apply an aspirin tablet directly to a canker sore and hold for 5-10 minutes twice a day. The pain will soon disappear, eventually along with the sore. For multiple sores, try crushing a tablet in a glass of water and holding the water in your mouth. Spit out afterwards (you don't want to swallow the canker toxins).

- **Alum:** Alum, which can be found in the spice rack of your grocery store, can be briefly applied to a canker sore 2-3 times a day to get rid of sores. It will hurt, and you will want to wash the bad taste out of your mouth, but it can be very effective.
- **Baking Soda:** Make a paste of baking soda and water, and then apply it to any canker sore. Leave it be for as long as possible. Reapply a few times a day and expect to be rid of the sore within a few days.
- **Salt:** If you can tolerate the brief increase in pain, a bit of salt dabbed on a canker sore or a warm saltwater mouthwash can get rid of a canker sore in a few applications.
- **Hydrogen Peroxide:** Dab a bit of hydrogen peroxide on a canker sore, or use a small bit of hydrogen peroxide as a mouthwash, to kill off whatever infection is creating the sores.
- **L-Lysine:** L-Lysine tablets taken twice a day can cure an attack of canker sores. Supplementing this essential amino acid seems to restore the body's ability to heal itself.
- **Toothpaste w/o SLS:** The abrasive nature of brushing your teeth can trigger a canker sore on its own. Worse yet, SLS (Sodium Lauryl Sulfite) is a common preservative that seems to be a further trigger. So be certain to choose a toothpaste free of SLS and you might stop your canker sore attacks.
- **Yogurt:** The active cultures in yogurt may be able to restore balance to the internal chemistry of your mouth, throat, and overall digestive system and thereby cure the canker sores. Simply eat yogurt containing active cultures once or twice a day.

MRSA

Multidrug-resistant Staphylococcus aureus (MRSA) is an umbrella term that designates any form of staph infection (a bacteria) that is resistant to a number of typical antibiotics, making it difficult to treat. MRSA initially looks like small red bumps akin to acne or spider bites, but it will progress into large, pus-filled boils.

BEST REMEDIES:
- **Turmeric:** Far and away the most popular boil remedy, turmeric is a powerful health aid (and a spice) from India. Drink one teaspoon of turmeric in water or milk 2-3 times a day until the boil has healed.
- **Garlic:** Eating a clove of raw garlic daily can help kill a staph infection from the inside. You can also crush the garlic into a paste and apply it to a boil for 10-20 minutes at a time, 2-3 times a day.

Muscle Cramps

Muscle cramps are the worst when they strike in the middle of the night, but they can be painful at any time. Most often caused by a blood deficiency or environmental factor, they can also be symptomatic of some conditions.

BEST REMEDIES:
- **Apple Cider Vinegar:** Add about one tablespoon of apple cider vinegar to a glass of water and drink straightaway. Relieves a cramped muscle in record time!
- **Pickle Juice:** Drinking a few ounces of pickle juice - you can take it straight from the jar - can stop a cramp fast and keep them from coming back anytime soon.
- **Banana:** Eating a banana is a long-standing home remedy for relieving muscle cramps, but there is good reason for that. Bananas are readily available and have a relatively large share of potassium—a mineral crucial to proper muscle function.

N

Nails, Fungus

Yellowed, thickened nails are the most obvious sign of a fungus infection around your finger or toenails. A small white or yellow spot underneath a nail may be the first sign of fungal infection.

BEST REMEDIES:
- **Apple Cider Vinegar:** A daily apple cider vinegar (ACV) tonic (up to two tablespoons of ACV in a tall glass of water) and daily ACV soak of the affected nails (mix water and ACV 2:1 in a basic and soak for 10-20 minutes) can kill nail fungus. Be aware that the ACV soak can further discolor the nails.
- **Oil of Oregano:** Used as directed internally and externally, oil of oregano can be a very effective anti-fungal, although it is a bit expensive. Mix with a kitchen oil to apply to the affected nail.
- **Lemongrass Essential Oil:** Lemongrass essential oil can be mixed with a kitchen oil (mix about 12 drops to an ounce of oil) and applied directly to the affected nail twice a day to kill off a fungal infection. You will need to reapply for several weeks until the infection is completely gone.
- **Hydrogen Peroxide:** Use a cotton swab to apply 3% hydrogen peroxide directly to the affected nail (not the skin!) twice a day to kill nail fungus within a couple of weeks.
- **Tea Tree Oil:** Use a cotton swab to apply tea tree oil directly to the affected nail 2-3 times a day for several weeks until the fungus is completely eradicated.
- **Distilled Vinegar:** Cheaper than apple cider vinegar, regular distilled vinegar works for many people to kill off a nail fungus infection. Simply mix water and white vinegar in a 2:1 solution (mostly water) and soak the

affected nails for 10-20 minutes once or twice daily until the infection clears. You can also dab vinegar directly on the infected nails.
- **Listerine:** Soak a cotton ball in Listerine and hold the cotton to the affected nail for at least 10-20 minutes once or twice a day. In 2-3 weeks, the infection should be eliminated and the nails on their way to recovery.
- **Iodine:** Apply iodine to the fungal infected nails and the skin around them once a day as an antifungal agent. Within a few weeks, the infection should be gone. Colorless iodine is available.

Nausea

Nausea and vomiting are common symptoms of a large number of illnesses and conditions. It may be an attempt to expel a pathogen or toxin, but nausea may also occur as a response to pain, due a loss of equilibrium, as 'morning sickness', in reaction to medications, etc.

BEST REMEDIES:
- **Alcohol Swabs:** Taking a quick sniff of an alcohol swab coated with isopropyl alcohol can quickly banish nausea for a number of people.
- **Baking Soda:** Add an eighth of a teaspoon of baking soda to a warm glass of water and sip slowly. The nausea should pass within a few minutes.

Neck, pain

Injury and damage to soft tissues are the most common causes of neck pain, but arthritis, degenerative disc disease, a herniated disc, and other more serious conditions are also a possibility.

BEST REMEDY:
- **Apple Cider Vinegar:** Soak a paper towel in apple cider vinegar and place it over the affected part of the neck, leaving it there for a couple of hours. People experience

dramatic relief in just one application, but it can be repeated later in the day.

Neck, stiff

If a stiff neck is accompanied by a fever, the sufferer should be checked out for meningitis, a serious condition. However, in most cases a stiff neck will pass within a few days. Muscle strains are a common cause, but holding your neck in an unnatural position for a period of time can also bring on the stiffness.

BEST REMEDIES:
- **Apple Cider Vinegar:** Soak a paper towel in apple cider vinegar and place it over the affected part of the neck, leaving it there for a couple of hours. People experience dramatic relief in just one application, but it can be repeated later in the day.
- **Arnica:** Arnica gel or oil can be massaged into a stiff neck or other weary or injured muscles to quickly relieve pain and swelling. Repeated use will speed healing, plus it's odorless and fairly easy to find.

Oral Herpes

Cold sores, caused by the herpes simplex virus, are fairly common but nonetheless irritating and embarrassing. We have found that they are triggered and exacerbated by artificial sweeteners. Yet one more reason to avoid them!

BEST REMEDIES:
- **Acetone Nail Polish Remover:** Use a cotton swab to apply a bit of acetone nail polish remover to a cold sore about once an hour until the cold sore is gone—often in a day or two!
- **Hydrogen Peroxide:** Dip a cotton swab in hydrogen peroxide and apply to any cold sore every few hours throughout the day to get rid of a cold sore within about three days.
- **Apple Cider Vinegar:** You'll feel a bit of a burning at first, but if you dab a bit of apple cider vinegar on a cold sore, it should dry out and disappear within about three days. Reapply about 4-5 times a day.
- **Ear Wax:** Odd but true! As soon as you get a cold sore tingle, apply a bit of your own earwax to the spot to stop the eruption from ever forming. Works even after the cold sore has formed. Leave it on, but don't lick your lips (yuck!).
- **L-Lysine:** Start taking the essential amino acid L-Lysine (in pill form) as soon as you feel a cold sore forming. You can reduce the number/size of cold stores or stop the outbreak entirely.
- **Garlic:** Cut a clove of garlic in small pieces and hold a piece to your cold sore for about ten minutes, 3-5 times a day (no more!) to dry out your cold sore and kill the virus at the same time.

- **Coconut Oil:** Adding up to a tablespoonful of cold pressed coconut oil to your daily diet (start with an eighth of a teaspoonful and increase slowly) can put an end to your cold sore attacks. For an active cold sore, try applying coconut oil directly to the sore a few times a day and leaving it there.

Ovarian Cysts

Many women have ovarian cysts without any problems from them, but for other women an ovarian cyst can cause pain, bleeding, and other issues. These cysts are simply fluids behind a thin wall within the ovary; however, their size can vary from very small to softball size or larger.

BEST REMEDY:
- **Beets, Molasses, and Aloe Vera:** Before any other meal each morning, eat this combination once a day. Mash 1-2 beet slices in a bowl, then add one tablespoon each of aloe vera juice and molasses. Eat this daily until the cysts have disappeared and symptoms have stopped.

Pain, severe

While pain is meant to alert the body to danger and prevent further harm, severe pain and chronic pain can be debilitating all by themselves. Injuries, nerve damage, degenerative conditions, neuropathy, backaches, and arthritis are just some of the many causes of chronic pain.

BEST REMEDIES:
- **Apple Cider Vinegar:** An apple cider vinegar (ACV) tonic can restore balance to your body's metabolism, relieving inflammation and improving overall systemic function to reduce pain symptoms. Take the ACV tonic three times a day with meals—one teaspoon of ACV in a large glass of water (honey optional). Increase the amount of ACV to 1-2 tablespoons per glass as your body tolerates it.
- **Turmeric:** Among other admirable qualities, turmeric is a strong anti-inflammatory. Add one teaspoonful each of turmeric powder and honey to a warm glass of milk (almond or rice will do as well as dairy) for daily use. Also available in pill form.
- **Blackstrap Molasses:** Nutrient and mineral-rich blackstrap molasses undergoes an additional refining step over the stuff you ordinarily find in the grocery store. Adding a daily tablespoon of blackstrap molasses to your diet can restore needed nutrients to your body, improving the body's functioning so that the source of pain can be eliminated. Many people like the taste of it in coffee!

Period Pain

While some cramping is normal for all women, dysmenorrhea, heavy bleeding, missed periods, extreme cramping, and other menstruation issues can make a woman's 'time of the month' unnecessarily challenging.

BEST REMEDIES:
- **Blackstrap Molasses:** Add 1 tsp to 1 Tbsp of blackstrap molasses (more concentrated than the kind you'll find on most grocery store shelves) to your daily diet. It's a strong taste, but you can combine it with many foods, and its rich mix of nutrients (and iron!) has brought many women dramatic relief.
- **Apple Cider Vinegar:** Many women have found quick relief from heavy bleeding, cramping, missed periods, and other menstruation concerns with the apple cider vinegar (ACV) tonic taken 1-3 times a day with meals. Mix 1 tsp - 2 Tbsp apple cider vinegar in a large glass of water, w/ or w/o honey, and sip slowly.

Phlebitis

An inflamed vein, called phlebitis, can be extremely uncomfortable. It can also be associated with Deep Vein Thrombosis, otherwise known as 'economy class syndrome'.

BEST REMEDY:
- **Lemon and Baking Soda:** Take the freshly squeezed juice of a lemon (or lime) and slowly add baking soda to the glass until the mixture stops fizzing, then add 4 oz. of water. Take twice a day, once in the morning and once before bedtime on an empty stomach.

Pink Eye

Conjunctivitis, better known as 'pink eye', is a viral infection that causes irritation, watering, reddening of the eyes, and a distinct pinkness of the eye's conjunctiva (the combined area at the edge of the eye and on the inside of the eyelid). A bacterial form is also possible.

BEST REMEDIES:

- **Apple Cider Vinegar:** Mix about two teaspoons of unpasteurized apple cider vinegar in a cup of water, then dip a cotton pad or soft cloth in it to wash the eyelid inside and out. You can place a few drops of the water mixture in the eye as well. Repeat every few hours until the conjunctivitis is all gone, usually 2-3 days. This mixture may burn a bit.
- **Green Tea Bags:** Put two green tea bags in a cup of hot water and allow the tea to brew and then cool somewhat, then apply each bag to an eye. Re-warm in the water and continue for about 10 minutes. Repeat every few hours until healed, usually 2-3 days.
- **Colloidal Silver:** Place a drop of colloidal silver in the affected eye 2-3 times a day until symptoms are gone.
- **Sea Salt:** Combine a tablespoon of sea salt in a cup of water and apply 2-3 drops to the corners of your eyes first thing in the morning and last thing at night.
- **Black Tea Bag:** Make a cup of black tea and allow it to cool a bit. Then apply the tea bag to the eye and keep it there for ten minutes or so. Repeat every few hours for the 1-3 days it will take to clear up the conjunctivitis.

Plantar Fasciitis

Heel spurs, calcified growths on the heel bone, are often accompanied by plantar fasciitis, a painful inflammation of the connective tissue supporting the arch of your foot. Most often, the pain is felt directly beneath the heel.

BEST REMEDY:

- **Apple Cider Vinegar Wrap:** Soak a cloth or bandage in apple cider vinegar and apply to the heel. You can leave it on for several hours, even wrap a plastic bag around heel and cloth to sleep with it at night. The pain should recede quickly and the underlying condition should be gone within a few weeks of daily treatment.

PMS

Premenstrual cramps, bloating, headaches, and other symptoms of PMS can make a woman's life miserable for a few days each month, but the right changes or additions to your diet can relieve or prevent PMS symptoms.

BEST REMEDY:

- **Apple Cider Vinegar:** What you need is the ACV Tonic! Mix 2 teaspoons of apple cider vinegar in 16 ounces of water that you'll sip throughout the day. You will be keeping your pH in a constant, alkalized state by sipping this highly diluted dosage. Usually 1-2 tall glasses of the concoction are all you'll need each day.

Poison Ivy

Oh, the scourge of poison ivy! The oozing rash, intense itch, and spreading contact dermatitis of poison ivy can expand from a small area of initial exposure to the plant (and its compound, urushiol) to cover large parts of the body and even become an internal infection.

BEST REMEDIES:

- **Jewel Weed:** Jewel Weed, sometimes known as Touch-Me-Not, is another plant that often grows beside poison ivy. Break the plant's stem and rub the escaping juices onto the poison ivy rash to clear up the blisters and relieve itching. Re-apply if it washes off. Jewelweed tincture is also available at health stores.
- **Fels-Naptha:** You will find this stuff in the laundry detergent section of your local grocery store. Ordinarily used to treat stains, you can rub the bar of soap on affected areas of the skin with cold water several times a day to relieve itching for hours and quickly dry up the blisters.

Prostate, enlarged

It is common for the prostate gland to become enlarged as a man ages. The prostate gland doesn't usually cause problems until later in life—it rarely causes symptoms before age 40. However, more than 50% of men in their sixties and as many as 90% in their seventies and eighties have some symptoms of an enlarged prostate.

BEST REMEDY:

- **Apple Cider Vinegar:** The ACV Tonic can help to restore the body's acid/alkaline balance and overall excretory health, reducing prostate issues. Mix 2 teaspoons of apple cider vinegar in 16 ounces of water that you'll sip throughout the day. You will be keeping your pH in a constant, alkalized state by sipping this highly diluted dosage. Usually 1-2 tall glasses of the concoction are all you'll need each day.

Psoriasis

The most obvious symptoms of psoriasis are the psoriatic plaques, inflamed areas of the skin exacerbated by excessive skin growth in the affected area. However, psoriasis is a disease (non-communicable) that can also affect the joints and nails.

BEST REMEDIES:

- **Apple Cider Vinegar:** Start with the ACV Tonic—Mix 2 teaspoons of apple cider vinegar in 16 ounces of water that you'll sip throughout the day. You will be keeping your pH in a constant, alkalized state by sipping this highly diluted dosage. Usually 1-2 tall glasses of the concoction are all you'll need each day. You can also use a cotton ball to apply apple cider vinegar directly to affected patches of skin, but beware of the sting.
- **Omega 3 Supplements:** Fish oil or flaxseed oil will provide your body with needed omega 3 fatty acids. Along with a host of other benefits, these omega 3's can improve skin nutrition and hydration. Just be careful that you get pharmaceutical grade fish oil if you choose fish over flaxseed, so as to avoid mercury and other heavy metal contaminants.

Q-R

RA

Rheumatoid Arthritis (RA) is an autoimmune disorder that primarily strikes the joints, resulting in intense pain and immobility. However, in addition to the body's attacking its own joints, RA also affects other bodily organs in a progressive disease.

BEST REMEDY:

- **Apple Cider Vinegar:** The ACV Tonic is the best natural remedy for RA, helping to reduce inflammation and build-up in the joints while improving overall health. Mix 2 teaspoons of apple cider vinegar in 16 ounces of water that you'll sip throughout the day. You will be keeping your pH in a constant, alkalized state by sipping this highly diluted dosage. Usually 1-2 tall glasses of the concoction are all you'll need each day.

Rash

A rash can take on any number of appearances and annoying characteristics – from the merely unsightly to the downright aggravating – and can be caused by a wide variety of infections, allergens, or wider medical conditions.

BEST REMEDIES:

- **Apple Cider Vinegar:** Dabbing undiluted apple cider vinegar on a rash can relieve itching and irritation quickly. The nutrients in unpasteurized ACV can also help to heal the skin while the acetic acid kills off opportunistic infections or even the agent causing the rash. Apply for a few minutes several times a day.
- **Coconut Oil:** Rub a bit of natural coconut oil into a rash – just like body lotion – and experience quick relief from

irritation. Often the rash soon disappears as well. Great for diaper rash!

Restless Legs Syndrome

RLS, or Restless Leg Syndrome, is most disturbing when trying to get to sleep but can strike during any period of relaxation. RLS sufferers report feeling irresistible urges to move the legs and odd sensations such as an itch or tickle. It is a neurological condition that often results in the person's legs jerking about, which can disrupt sleep.

BEST REMEDIES:
- **Bar of Soap:** Some remedies are as inexplicable as they are effective! For this one, take a bar of Ivory soap (it can stay in its wrapper or go into a sock) and bring it to bed with you. You can hold onto it, put it at the foot of the bed, or alongside you somewhere between the knees and hips.
- **Baking Soda:** Half an hour before bed, mix one-quarter teaspoon of baking soda in a small glass of water and drink. Within about 20 minutes, your legs should be at ease.

Rheumatoid Arthritis

Rheumatoid Arthritis (RA) is an autoimmune disorder that primarily strikes the joints, resulting in intense pain and immobility. However, in addition to the body's attacking its own joints, RA also affects other bodily organs in a progressive disease.

BEST REMEDY:
- **Apple Cider Vinegar:** The ACV Tonic is the best natural remedy for RA, helping to reduce inflammation and build-up in the joints while improving overall health. Mix 2 teaspoons of apple cider vinegar in 16 ounces of water that you'll sip throughout the day. You will be keeping your pH in a constant, alkalized state by sipping this highly diluted dosage. Usually 1-2 tall glasses of the concoction are all you'll need each day.

Ringing of the Ears

Tinnitus is a symptom of many conditions. The tinnitus sufferer "hears" ringing in the ears where there is no external sound to cause it. This may be temporary and the result of some aural damage, such as a loud concert, or it may be a life-long condition without clear cause or remedy. Medications and age-related hearing loss can result in tinnitus, but loud noises are the most common cause.

BEST REMEDY:

- **Apple Cider Vinegar:** Daily use of the ACV Tonic might be able to reduce the ringing in your ears. Mix 2 teaspoons of apple cider vinegar in 16 ounces of water that you'll sip throughout the day. You will be keeping your pH in a constant, alkalized state by sipping this highly diluted dosage. Usually 1-2 tall glasses of the concoction are all you'll need each day.

Ringworm

Also known as Tinea, Ringworm is a contagious fungal infection that can affect the scalp, body, feet, and nails. Despite its name, it has nothing to do with worms! The name comes from a characteristic red ring that appears on the infected person's skin.

BEST REMEDIES:

- **Apple Cider Vinegar:** Two to three times a day, use a cotton swab to apply apple cider vinegar directly to the ringworm scab. Do not wash off. You should see results within a couple of days and be rid of ringworm within a couple of weeks.
- **Bleach:** Dilute one part bleach in ten parts water and apply to any patches of ringworm 2-4 times a day to clear up ringworm within several days. Bleach is a strong chemical agent, so always be careful in your dilution and application!

Rosacea

Rosacea is an inflammatory skin disease that causes facial redness. It affects mostly adults, usually people with fair skin, between the ages of 30 and 60, more commonly in women. Left untreated, rosacea tends to worsen over time. However, in many sufferers, rosacea is cyclic, so your skin may flare up for a period of time and then lessen before flaring up again.

BEST REMEDIES:
- **Apple Cider Vinegar:** Topical and internal use of apple cider vinegar (ACV) can cure rosacea in a few weeks. Use a cotton swab to apply undiluted ACV to affected patches of skin 2-3 times a day. Additionally, take the ACV tonic 1-3 times a day with meals—one teaspoon of ACV in a large glass of water (honey optional). Increase the amount of ACV to 1-2 tablespoons per glass as your body tolerates it.
- **Tea Tree Oil:** Apply a drop or two of tea tree oil to a moistened cotton swab and wipe it across affected skin twice a day.

S

Scabies

Scabies is a contagious disorder of the skin caused by very small, wingless insects or mites. The female insect digs into the skin where she lays 1 - 3 eggs daily. If untreated, the female will continue to lay eggs for about five weeks. A very small, hard to see, zigzag blister usually marks the trail of the insect as she lays her eggs. More obvious signs are an intense itching (especially at night) and a red rash.

BEST REMEDIES:
- **Borax and Hydrogen Peroxide:** Draw a hot bath. Add one cup of borax detergent and one half cup of peroxide to the bathwater and bathe as usual. The itching should stop immediately, and you should see improvement within a couple of days. Repeat daily as needed.
- **Bleach:** Dilute one part bleach in four parts water and spray onto the affected skin once or twice a day. Bleach is a strong chemical agent, so always be careful in your dilution and application!

Scalp Infections

Ringworm is the most common scalp infection, resulting in itchy, red rings of infected skin. The hair may fall out in circular patches.

BEST REMEDY:
- **Hydrogen Peroxide and Apple Cider Vinegar:** Mix one part hydrogen peroxide, one part apple cider vinegar, and ten parts water. Use this solution just as you would a shampoo, massaging into the scalp and hair. Leave it in place for a minute or two before washing out. This should kill off most scalp infections (including ringworm) within a week's worth of applications.

Scalp Ringworm

Also known as Tinea, Ringworm is a contagious fungal infection that can affect the scalp, body, feet, and nails. Despite its name, it has nothing to do with worms! The name comes from a characteristic red ring that appears on the infected person's skin. On the scalp, ringworm begins as a small pimple that becomes larger, leaving scaly patches of temporary baldness. Infected hairs become brittle and break off easily.

BEST REMEDIES:
- **Apple Cider Vinegar:** Two to three times a day, use a cotton swab to apply apple cider vinegar directly to the ringworm scab. Do not wash off. You should see results within a couple of days and be rid of ringworm within a couple of weeks.
- **Bleach:** Dilute one part bleach in ten parts water and apply to any patches of ringworm 2-4 times a day to clear up ringworm within several days.

Scar

Where a wound has damaged the skin extensively, a scar may form as part of the healing process. This tougher, fibrous form of skin tissue can disfigure the skin and be a different coloration.

BEST REMEDY:
- **Vitamin E:** Vigorously massaging Vitamin E oil into scar tissue several times a day can slowly but very effectively restore the skin to its original condition.

Schizophrenia

Schizophrenia is a psychiatric disorder that affects over two million Americans. Characterized by distortions in thinking & perception – and often accompanied by emotions inappropriate to the given situation – researchers believe it is caused by an imbalance of key chemicals in the brain.

BEST REMEDY:
- **Gluten-Free Diet:** Even psychiatrists are now considering the idea of recommending a gluten-free diet to help patients get control of a schizophrenic condition. Some people have been able to go off their medications thanks to this dietary change!

Sciatica

If damaged or pinched, the sciatic nerve running from the lower back down through the back of the leg can create pain, tingling, numbness and other symptoms.

BEST REMEDIES:
- **Candied Ginger:** Candied ginger or crystallized ginger can be an easy and tasty remedy for sciatic pain. Eat a couple of pieces a day, maybe more on the first day, for lasting relief.
- **Tennis Shoes:** This one is fascinating! Take a tennis shoe and set it down on a firm chair with the heel facing forward, then sit on the shoe, rather as if it were a bike seat. You'll experience some discomfort at first, but you should find lasting relief within 20 minutes or more.

Seborrheic Dermatitis (Dandruff)

The itchy scalp of a dandruff condition and the embarrassing white flakes compete to see which can be the worse symptom of this common condition.

BEST REMEDIES:
- **Apple Cider Vinegar:** Dilute apple cider vinegar 1:1 with water and then use just like a shampoo to clean your hair and scalp. Should cure the itch instantly and get rid of dandruff within several days worth of applications.
- **Apple Cider Vinegar and Hydrogen Peroxide:** Combine 1 part apple cider vinegar and 1 part Hydrogen

Peroxide with 10 parts water. Use like a shampoo and rinse after the mixture has set for a few minutes. Should clear up dandruff in 2-3 days.

- **Omega 3 Supplements:** Fish oil or flaxseed oil will provide your body with needed omega 3 fatty acids. Along with a host of other benefits, these omega 3's can improve scalp nutrition and hydration. Just be careful that you get pharmaceutical grade fish oil if you choose fish over flaxseed, so as to avoid mercury and other heavy metal contaminants.

Severe Dandruff

The itchy scalp of a dandruff condition and the embarrassing white flakes compete to see which can be the worse symptom of this common condition.

BEST REMEDIES:
- **Apple Cider Vinegar:** Dilute apple cider vinegar 1:1 with water and then use just like a shampoo to clean your hair and scalp. Should cure the itch instantly and get rid of dandruff within several days worth of applications.
- **Apple Cider Vinegar and Hydrogen Peroxide:** Combine 1 part apple cider vinegar and 1 part Hydrogen Peroxide with 10 parts water. Use like a shampoo and rinse after the mixture has set for a few minutes. Should clear up dandruff in 2-3 days.

Severe Contact Dermatitis

Dermatitis, a general inflammation of the skin, can take many forms—from contact dermatitis and eczema to perioral and discoid dermatitis. It can present itself as an irritation, rash, or even blisters.

BEST REMEDIES:
- **Apple Cider Vinegar:** Apply a 50/50 concentration of apple cider vinegar and water to a rash and then rinse

off after several minutes. Do this twice a day until the dermatitis heals.

- **Grapefruit Seed Extract:** Add 8-20 drops of grapefruit seed extract to 4 oz. of water and drink twice daily. You can also dab the mixture on the rash and then rinse off after a few minutes.
- **Coconut Oil:** Apply a small amount of coconut oil to any rash several times a day, just like lotion, to stop the irritation and cure most dermatitis within a few days.

Shingles

Shingles (also known as Herpes Zoster or the varicella-zoster virus) is a painful, blistering rash caused by the same virus as chickenpox. Someone with shingles may feel unwell and develop a localized area of pain a few days before the rash appears. The rash starts off as red spots, which quickly turn into blisters. Shingles affects only a limited area of skin, yet the pain from these blisters can be intense.

BEST REMEDY:

- **Apple Cider Vinegar:** Topical and internal use of apple cider vinegar (ACV) can reduce shingles symptoms and potentially cure the condition. Use a cotton swab to apply undiluted ACV to affected patches of skin 2-3 times a day. Additionally, take the ACV tonic 3 times a day with meals—one teaspoon each of ACV and honey in a large glass of water. Increase the amount of ACV to 1-2 tablespoons per glass as your body tolerates it.

Sinus Congestion

Sinus congestion and congestion in the throat and lungs can be debilitating and even dangerous. Mucus/phlegm plays a role in preventing illness, but too much of it can be just as much of a problem, not to mention the discomfort.

BEST REMEDIES:

- **Jean's Famous Tomato Tea:** Outrageously popular, this simple home remedy from our friend Jeannie Woolhiser of Wisconsin clears sinus congestion almost immediately and can bring a quick end to a cold. Mix and heat the following recipe on the stove, then drink and inhale the steam (be careful!) until after your symptoms have disappeared.

  ### TOMATO TEA RECIPE
  2 cups tomato juice
  2-3 cloves garlic crushed (use more if you can)
  2 T lemon juice
  Hot sauce (the more the better, as much as you can handle)

- **Apple Cider Vinegar:** The apple cider vinegar tonic, taken two-three times a day, can quickly break up congestion and improve other cold and flu symptoms as well. Add one tablespoon each apple cider vinegar and honey to a tall glass of warm water, and sip.
- **Oil Pulling:** The Ayurvedic tradition of oil pulling can remove toxins from the body and clear up congestion as well. Before brushing your teeth and with an empty stomach, take one Tbsp of oil into your mouth and swish it around for 10-20 minutes until the oil has turned milky white. Then spit out. Most any food oil will do, but sesame and sunflower oils are traditional and the most popular.
- **Neti Pot:** The traditional neti pot can be an excellent general health tool, but it is especially effective at cleaning out the sinuses and relieving congestion. Check out EarthClinic.com or a trusted source on the proper use of neti pots.
- **Steaming:** Drape a towel over your head and neck, then carefully hold your face over a steaming pot of water (not too hot!). Breathe in the steam for several minutes, and repeat throughout the day. For added effect, try adding

lavender oil, a tablespoon of apple cider vinegar, or some essential oils from the mint family for even greater effect.

Sinus Infections

Sinus infections, resulting in sinusitis, are miserable affairs with full, inflamed sinus cavities causing facial pain, headache, inner ear problems, thick nasal discharge, and other symptoms. It can be caused by a virus, bacteria, or fungus and often is preceded by a respiratory infection.

BEST REMEDIES:
- **Apple Cider Vinegar:** The apple cider vinegar tonic, taken two-three times a day, can quickly break up congestion and improve other cold and flu symptoms as well. Add one tablespoon each apple cider vinegar and honey to a tall glass of warm water, and sip.
- **Saline Rinse:** Mix a half-teaspoon of sea salt in a cup of warm water, then irrigate the nose with a nasal spray bottle or neti pot.
- **Hydrogen Peroxide and Sea Salt:** In six ounces of warm water, mix a teaspoon of sea salt and a half-teaspoon of hydrogen peroxide. Use this solution to irrigate the nostrils with a nasal sprayer or neti pot.
- **Cayenne Pepper:** Take a small pinch of cayenne pepper powder and snort it up each nostril. It may hurt a bit at first, but your sinuses will quickly drain.
- **Steaming:** Drape a towel over your head and neck, then carefully hold your face over a steaming pot of water (not too hot!). Breathe in the steam for several minutes, and repeat throughout the day. For added effect, try adding lavender oil, a tablespoon of apple cider vinegar, or some essential oils from the mint family for even greater effect.
- **Hydrogen Peroxide:** Mix four parts water with one part hydrogen peroxide, then irrigate the nose with a nasal spray bottle or neti pot.
- **Grapefruit Seed Extract:** Add 4 drops of grapefruit seed extract and a quarter tsp of sea salt to 8oz of warm

water, then irrigate the nose with a nasal spray bottle or neti pot.

- **Neti Pot:** The traditional neti pot can be an excellent general health tool, but it is especially effective at cleaning out the sinuses and relieving congestion. Check out EarthClinic.com or a trusted source on the proper use of neti pots.
- **Oil Pulling:** The Ayurvedic tradition of oil pulling can remove toxins from the body and clear up congestion as well. Before brushing your teeth and with an empty stomach, take one Tbsp of oil into your mouth and swish it around for 10-20 minutes until the oil has turned milky white. Then spit out. Most any food oil will do, but sesame and sunflower oils are traditional and the most popular.
- **Oil of Oregano:** Put a couple of drops of oregano oil beneath your tongue to relieve sinus pressure. You can also add a few drops to a steaming pot of water and drape a cloth over your head and neck to breathe in the vapors.

Skin, Acne

Common acne is generally most acute in teenagers but can still be an occasional or constant problem for adults as well. The face, back, and chest are most commonly affected.

BEST REMEDIES:
- **Apple Cider Vinegar:** A daily ACV tonic (1 tsp - 2 Tbsp apple cider vinegar in a large glass of water, w/ or w/o honey) can clarify the skin and give it a healthy glow. A couple of teaspoons of ACV diluted in a cup of water can be used as a skin toner.
- **Hydrogen Peroxide:** Dip a cotton ball in hydrogen peroxide, then dab it all over the affected skin. Hold the cotton ball to existing blemishes for a couple of minutes for deeper treatment.
- **Coconut Oil:** Using coconut oil as a daily moisturizer on the affected areas of the skin can clear up breakouts and

improve the overall look of your skin.

- **Tea Tree Oil:** Use a cotton swab to dab tea tree oil on existing acne a few times a day to dry out the oily skin and clear up the blemish.
- **Urine:** Soak a cotton ball or pad in your own urine (the morning's first urine is most effective) and use it to scrub the affected areas of the skin.
- **Garlic:** Add raw garlic to your daily diet, and its antibacterial allicin compound will kill off the bacteria that cause acne on your skin.
- **Lemons:** Use a bit of lemon juice like a toner to clear away excess oils and clarify your skin. Feel free to dilute in a bit of water as well if the lemon has a bite to it.
- **Baking Soda:** Make a paste of a bit of baking soda and water, then use as a facial scrub. For more extensive body acne, put two tablespoons of baking soda in your bathwater.
- **Aloe Vera:** Apply aloe vera gel directly to your skin 2-3 times a day to clean and dry up excess oils on your skin.

Skin, Beautiful

The first step to beautiful skin is to remove makeup, oil, and environmental contaminants from your skin. Exfoliation is the next essential step, in order to remove dead skin cells from the skin's surface. A few of our reader-recommended home remedies can make the whole process more effective.

BEST REMEDIES:
- **Apple Cider Vinegar:** The ACV Tonic is just the thing to get healthy skin, starting from the inside! Mix 2 teaspoons of apple cider vinegar in 16 ounces of water that you'll sip throughout the day. You will be keeping your pH in a constant, alkalized state by sipping this highly diluted dosage. Usually 1-2 tall glasses of the concoction are all you'll need each day. You can also use a cotton swab

dabbed in ACV as a facial wash, cleansing and restoring the skin's naturally acidic mantle.

- **Baking Soda:** About once a week, mix a bit of baking soda with enough water to make a paste and gently scrub this into your skin. Baking soda makes an excellent exfoliant and keeps pathogens under control.
- **Coconut Oil:** Use coconut oil as you would a moisturizing skin lotion to tighten up the skin and give it a healthy glow. An excellent beauty care product!
- **Brown Sugar Scrub:** This occasional body scrub is all natural, inexpensive, and delightfully effective! Mix a quarter-cup of brown sugar with one tablespoon of honey and one teaspoon of apple cider vinegar. Gently scrub into the face and any skin that needs to be exfoliated and restored.

Skin Infections (cysts, boils)

Boils and cysts seem to be increasingly common. Usually the result of a staph infection, this form of folliculitis results in an accumulation of pus and a hard core at the center of the boil that will need to be removed.

BEST REMEDIES:
- **Turmeric:** Far and away the most popular boil remedy, turmeric is a powerful health aid (and a spice) from India. Drink one teaspoon of turmeric in water 2-3 times a day until the boil has healed.
- **Baking Soda:** A paste of baking soda and water can be applied to a boil and left on to draw out the infection and dry out the boil.
- **Garlic:** Eating a clove of raw garlic daily can help kill a staph infection from the inside. You can also crush the garlic into a paste and apply it to a boil for 10-20 minutes at a time, 2-3 times a day.
- **Iodine:** Apply iodine to a boil and the area immediately around it to stop a boil and prevent the staph infection from spreading.

- **Apple Cider Vinegar:** Dab a cotton ball in apple cider vinegar and tape it to the boil, then replace it twice a day. Also, try the ACV tonic (1tsp-2Tbsp apple cider vinegar in a tall glass of water, natural sweetener optional).

Skin, Itchy

Dry and itchy skin is about as common a condition as you can get, though drier climates and colder winter seasons can exacerbate the problem. Too much sun exposure, change in diet, medications, and any number of other influences can cause temporary itching as well.

BEST REMEDY:
- **Apple Cider Vinegar:** Soak a cloth in apple cider vinegar and place it on the itchy skin for 15 minutes or more to soothe itchy skin. The vinegar's nutrients and antibiotic potency can potentially remedy the underlying cause, in addition.

Skin Tags

Skin tags are benign tumors that typically form in skin creases such as the neck and groin, though they may also appear on the face or other areas. They are harmless but can be painful to remove.

BEST REMEDIES:
- **Iodine:** Apply iodine directly to the skin tag, taking care to avoid healthy skin. Apply once or twice a day, expecting to see it fall off within several days time.
- **String:** Use a string of cotton or dental floss to tie a tight loop around the base of the skin tag to slowly cut off the supply of blood to the tag. It will fall off on its own in a couple of days.
- **Apple Cider Vinegar:** Dampen a cotton ball with apple cider vinegar and apply to the skin tag. Rub the tag with the cotton ball for a few minutes twice a day for a few days until the tag disappears or falls off.

Sleep, Poor Quality

The inability to fall asleep or stay asleep, no matter the cause, is called insomnia. Pain is the most frequent cause but medications, stress, and environmental changes are among the very many other causes.

BEST REMEDIES:

- **Apple Cider Vinegar:** Restoring your body's pH and nutritive balances might be all you need for a good night's sleep. Try adding an apple cider vinegar (ACV) tonic to your daily routine—Mix 2 teaspoons of apple cider vinegar in 16 ounces of water that you'll sip throughout the day. You will be keeping your pH in a constant, alkalized state by sipping this highly diluted dosage. Usually 1-2 tall glasses of the concoction are all you'll need each day.
- **Ear Plugs:** Blocking out the distracting sounds of the world can be the easiest way to get some much-needed sleep.
- **Melatonin:** Melatonin tablets, taken as directed, are a popular natural remedy for sleeplessness. It is a hormone that naturally occurs in the human body, helping to regulate the circadian (and thus sleep) rhythms.

Snoring

Generally, when it comes to snoring we pity the person "sleeping" next to the snorer, but the person who snores is likely losing out on quality sleep as well. Snoring can also be an indicator of other sleep or general health issues.

BEST REMEDY:

- **Apple Cider Vinegar:** Adding the ACV Tonic to your daily diet can remedy imbalances in your metabolic systems that may be leading to your snoring. Mix 2 teaspoons of apple cider vinegar in 16 ounces of water that you'll sip throughout the day. You will be keeping your pH in a constant, alkalized state by sipping this highly diluted dosage. Usually 1-2 tall glasses of the concoction are all you'll need each day.

Solar Keratosis

A solar keratosis is a small bump that develops on the skin. It is caused by excessive exposure to the sun over a period of time. One or more bumps may develop. The size of each bump can range from the size of a pinhead to 2-3 cm in diameter! It can be the same color as your skin – light, dark, pink, red – or a combo of these colors, and may have a yellow-white crust or feel rough and dry.

BEST REMEDY:
- **Apple Cider Vinegar:** Use a cotton ball to apply a bit of apple cider vinegar (ACV) directly to the affected skin 2-3 times a day. Supplement with a daily ACV Tonic—Take one teaspoon of ACV (honey optional) and mix it in a large glass of water. Drink with breakfast or each meal of the day. Increase the ACV in each glass to as much as 2 tablespoons.

Sore Throat

A sore throat is an infection of either viral or bacterial origin. It is most commonly caused by a contagious viral infection (such as the flu, cold, or mononucleosis), although more serious throat infections can be caused by a bacterial infection (such as strep, mycoplasma, or hemophilus). Bacterial sore throats respond well to antibiotics while viral infections do not.

BEST REMEDIES:
- **Cayenne:** Far and away the most popular sore throat remedy. Add a teaspoon of powdered cayenne pepper to a glass of warm water and repeatedly gargle with it. Sore throat pain vanishes, and other cold-like symptoms improve as well! (If your lips are raw, put on a little chapstick first to protect them.)
- **Apple Cider Vinegar:** Add 1-2 tablespoons of apple cider vinegar and some honey to a small glass of warm water and drink the mixture to soothe a sore throat and kill off an infection.

- **Pickle Juice Brine:** Drink and/or gargle with a couple of tablespoons of pickle juice to get the combined effects of salt and vinegar to soothe and cure your sore throat!
- **Salt Water Gargle:** Mix 3 teaspoons of salt in 2 cups of warm water and gargle with the mixture, spitting out and repeating several times.
- **Hot Sauce:** Add 5-6 drops of hot sauce to a glass of warm water and gargle and/or drink the mixture repeatedly to soothe and cure a sore throat. You can also add hot sauce to soups or other hot drinks.
- **Hydrogen Peroxide:** Dilute one part hydrogen peroxide in four parts water and use this solution as a gargle. DO NOT SWALLOW! Repeat several times.
- **Ginger:** Try out this excellent ginger tea for sore throats! Grate 1.5 tablespoons of fresh ginger into a cup, add a tablespoon of lemon or lime juice, and one teaspoon of honey then fill the mug with boiling water. Stir and allow to steep, then drink. Delicious and effective!
- **Lemon:** Squeeze the juice of an entire lemon into a mug of hot water and sweeten with honey. Drink to soothe and cure most sore throats. Not good for strep throat.

Spider Bites

Earth Clinic Warning: People are frequently mistaking MRSA-related boils for spider bites. Turns out that some doctors are making the same misdiagnosis as well! If you are not 100% sure that you were bitten by a spider, please make sure to take a look at our entry on Boils.

BEST REMEDIES:
- **Baking Soda:** Make a thick paste out of baking soda and water. Apply this to the spider bite and allow to dry. Once it has brushed off, reapply several times throughout the day to reduce the swelling and pain.
- **Salt:** Salt or saline can quickly reduce the pain and swelling of a spider bite. Either mix ample salt with water in a basin to soak the affected skin, or mix salt in a bit of water and

apply the paste to the wound and cover with a band-aid. Reapply as necessary.

Splinters

How do you remove a deeply-seated splinter from your finger or another body part? A few clever home remedies can make the process easier and perhaps prevent infection as well. Some splinter remedies work on cactus needles and other similar "stickers" as well.

BEST REMEDY:
- **White Vinegar:** Here's a clever home remedy. Soak the finger or other body part containing the sliver in a basin of white vinegar for several minutes. The wood or other material (cactus needles too!) may "leap" out on its own, or a little pressure will cause even deeply seated splinters to pop out enough to grab them.

Spurs, Heel

Heel spurs, calcified growths on the heel bone, are often accompanied by plantar fasciitis, a painful inflammation of the connective tissue supporting the arch of your foot. Most often, the pain is felt directly beneath the heel.

BEST REMEDY:
- **Apple Cider Vinegar Wrap:** Soak a cloth or bandage in apple cider vinegar and apply to the heel. You can leave it on for several hours, or even wrap a plastic bag around heel and cloth to sleep with it at night. The pain should recede quickly and the underlying condition should be gone within a few weeks of daily treatment.

Staph

Boils seem to be increasingly common. Usually the result of a staph (bacterial) infection, this form of folliculitis results in an accumulation of pus and a hard core at the center of the boil that will need to be removed. Multi-drug-resistant Staphylococcus aureus (MRSA) is an umbrella term that designates any form of staph infection that is resistant to a number of typical antibiotics.

BEST REMEDIES:
- **Turmeric:** Far and away the most popular staph remedy, turmeric is a powerful health aid (and a spice) from India. Drink one teaspoon of turmeric in water or milk 2-3 times a day until the boil has healed.
- **Garlic:** Eating a clove of raw garlic daily can help kill a staph infection from the inside. You can also crush the garlic into a paste and apply it to a boil for 10-20 minutes at a time, 2-3 times a day.

Stiff Neck

If a stiff neck is accompanied by a fever, the sufferer should be checked out for meningitis, a serious condition. However, in most cases a stiff neck will pass within a few days. Muscle strains are a common cause, but holding your neck in an unnatural position for a period of time can also bring on the stiffness.

BEST REMEDY:
- **Apple Cider Vinegar:** Soak a paper towel in apple cider vinegar and place it over the affected part of the neck, leaving it there for a couple of hours. People experience dramatic relief in just one application, but it can be repeated later in the day.

Stomach Ache and Issues

How do you cure a stomachache? A couple of home remedies rise above the rest as natural stomach ache cures, whether the cause be food poisoning, illness, or something else. A stomachache may or may not be associated with vomiting or nausea. Some stomach aches, particularly acute abdominal pain, can be a symptom of more serious conditions and should be addressed promptly.

BEST REMEDY:
- **Apple Cider Vinegar:** For food poisoning or intense stomach ache you can drink 1-2 tablespoons of apple cider vinegar (ACV) straight. However, in most cases it is enough to mix 2 teaspoons of apple cider vinegar in 16 ounces of water that you'll sip throughout the day.

Strep Throat

In the absence of a cough or cold, a sudden and severe sore throat may be a streptococcal or strep throat infection, a potentially serious condition that should be examined by a physician. However, a few at-home remedies can help in healing and reduce sore throat symptoms.

BEST REMEDIES:
- **Cayenne:** Far and away the most popular sore throat remedy. Add a teaspoon of powdered cayenne pepper to a glass of warm water and repeatedly gargle with it. Sore throat pain vanishes, and other cold-like symptoms improve as well! (If your lips are raw, put on a little chapstick first to protect them.)
- **Apple Cider Vinegar:** Add 1-2 tablespoons of apple cider vinegar and some honey to a small glass of warm water and drink the mixture to soothe a sore throat and kill off a strep infection.
- **Apple Cider Vinegar and Cayenne:** Mix one-half tablespoon of powdered cayenne pepper, 1 tablespoon of apple cider vinegar, and 1 tablespoon of honey or natural maple syrup together in a small glass of warm water. Sip and swallow until your symptoms are gone.
- **Garlic:** Eating (lots of) raw garlic or steeping garlic in warm water and drinking this "tea" can kill off a staph infection and relieve sore throat symptoms.

Sty

A sty is an acute infection or inflammation of the secretion glands of the eyelids. It results from blocked glands within the eyelid. When the gland is blocked, oil produced by the gland can back up through the wall of the gland, forming a lump. This lump can be red, painful, and nodular.

BEST REMEDIES:
- **Gold Wedding Band:** Another fascinatingly odd but exceedingly effective remedy! Take a gold wedding ring and rub it against the sty for about five minutes. Repeat a few times throughout the day. People report overnight cures.
- **Baby Shampoo:** Use a bit of baby shampoo a few times a day to wash out the area around the sty. The sty should disappear within a day or two.
- **Green Tea Bags:** Put a green tea bag in a cup of hot water and allow the tea to brew and then cool somewhat, then apply the bag to the affected eye. Re-warm in the water and continue for about 10 minutes. Repeat every few hours until healed, usually in a day or two.

Sunburn

Too much exposure to the ultraviolet light in sunlight or solar lamps can lead to a sunburn, a painful burn that will appear reddened, will be warm, and could be blistered. It may be accompanied by dizziness, fatigue, and dehydration and can lead to skin cancer over time.

BEST REMEDIES:
- **Apple Cider Vinegar:** Soak a cotton ball in apple cider vinegar and apply it to the burn to experience quick relief. Kills potential pathogens that could infect an open blister as well. The apple cider vinegar will soothe the skin and help it return to its normal condition more quickly.
- **Coconut Oil:** Use coconut oil just like lotion after a sunburn to soothe the skin and help restore it to health

more quickly. Apply once or twice a day.
- **Aloe Vera:** Aloe vera applied directly from a broken stem of the plant (or commercial aloe vera gel) will soothe and protect sunburned skin for immediate relief.

Swollen Lymph Nodes

Swollen lymph nodes are a common indication of some infection or illness in the body, though the infection can also strike the lymphatic system itself.

BEST REMEDY:
- **Apple Cider Vinegar:** To reduce the swelling lymph nodes, try an ACV tonic—one tablespoon of apple cider vinegar (ACV) in a large glass of water (honey optional).

T

Teeth, Stained

Looking for a safe home remedy to help you quickly whiten teeth or clean up stained teeth? At least one very effective natural remedy exists to get rid of tan or brown stains on teeth from coffee, tea, cigarettes, or just the passage of time.

BEST REMEDY:

- **Hydrogen Peroxide:** Hydrogen peroxide is a mild bleaching agent. Pour out about a tablespoon of 3% hydrogen peroxide and hold it in your mouth for several minutes, gently swishing the solution across your teeth to significantly whiten your teeth. For occasional use.

Throwing Up, Severe

Can't stop throwing up? We have one very fast-working Ayurvedic remedy involving onions and peppermint tea, with a couple of other remedies thrown in for good measure!

BEST REMEDIES:

- **Black Tea:** Brew a cup of black tea using two tea bags to create an extra strong cup of tea (add a teaspoon of honey, if you like). Within a few minutes of sipping the tea, your nausea should vanish.
- **Honey:** Eating a teaspoon of honey can stop nausea and vomiting in no time at all. Feel free to also add a bit of honey to food as you first begin to eat again afterwards to help the foods go down.
- **Onion Juice:** Prepare peppermint tea and allow to cool while you grate an onion. Squeeze the pulp through cheesecloth to make 1 tablespoon of Fresh Onion Juice. Hold your nose and swallow the onion juice, then follow with just 1

tablespoon of peppermint tea. Wait ten minutes. Take another tablespoon of peppermint tea. Wait 15 minutes. This remedy should stop vomiting within 15 minutes. The peppermint tea additionally helps to re-hydrate you.

Thyroid Issues

Hypothyroidism, a lack of certain hormones due to a low-functioning thyroid gland, can be the result of a number of conditions. It can have a number of early symptoms including fatigue, cold intolerance, constipation, thin and brittle fingernails, paleness, itchy skin, and weight gain. Its opposite, hyperthyroidism, can result in overproduction of hormones and create symptoms of jitteriness, insomnia, heart conditions, etc.

BEST REMEDIES:
- **Iodine:** Lugol's iodine, SSKI, or kelp supplements (taken as directed) can restore proper thyroid functioning for those with both hyperthyroidism and hypothyroidism.
- **Coconut Oil:** Add up to a tablespoon of coconut oil to your daily diet to get the general health benefits of this remarkable dietary aid and to improve thyroid function.

Tinea Capitis

Tinea capitis, also known as scalp ringworm, is the most common scalp infection, resulting in itchy, red rings of infected skin. The hair may fall out in circular patches.

BEST REMEDY:
- **Hydrogen Peroxide and Apple Cider Vinegar:** Mix one part hydrogen peroxide, one part apple cider vinegar, and ten parts water. Use this solution just as you would a shampoo, massaging into the scalp and hair. Leave it in place for a minute or two before washing out. This should kill off most scalp infections (including ringworm) within a week's worth of applications.

Tinnitus

Tinnitus is a symptom of many conditions. The tinnitus sufferer "hears" ringing in the ears where there is no external sound to cause it. This may be temporary and the result of some aural damage (such as a loud concert) or it may be a life-long condition without clear cause or remedy. Medications and age-related hearing loss can result in tinnitus, but loud noises are the most common cause.

BEST REMEDY:
- **Apple Cider Vinegar:** Daily use of the ACV Tonic might reduce the ringing in your ears. Mix 2 teaspoons of apple cider vinegar in 16 ounces of water that you'll sip throughout the day. You will be keeping your pH in a constant, alkalized state by sipping this highly diluted dosage. Usually 1-2 tall glasses of the concoction are all you'll need each day.

Tongue - White Coating

There are several possibilities for what causes a white coating on the tongue. The most common cause of a white coating is a candidal infection, thrush, which is caused by fungus. A white coating can also simply be the buildup of dead cells on the tongue. Finally, a white coating on the tongue may be caused by dehydration! Simply drinking more water will remedy this condition, so we suggest you try this first for a week or two and see if it makes a difference.

BEST REMEDY:
- **Salt:** Take sea salt or kosher salt and mix salt water to use as a mouthwash (try one teaspoon salt to a cup of water). For tough cases, follow up by placing salt directly on the tongue and holding it there for a few minutes before spitting out. Or put salt on your toothbrush and brush your tongue with it.

Toothache

Toothache can have many causes, some more severe than others, but in most cases the sufferer will have to deal with tooth pain at least for awhile before a dentist or orthodontist can deal with the essential cause of the pain. That's where natural remedies come in most handily!

BEST REMEDIES:

- **Garlic:** For toothache or a developing abscess, take a clove of garlic, place it on the affected tooth, and gently bite down on it so that the garlic juices begin to spread over the area. Pain may increase at first but should soon subside entirely. Garlic's sulfur and other components may be able to kill off the infection entirely.
- **Cloves:** Clove oil is a powerful anesthetic. Just a couple of drops on an aching tooth can instantly stop the pain. Repeat as necessary.
- **Oil Pulling:** The ancient practice of oil pulling is finding renewed fame for its ability to pull toxins out of the body. It may not relieve pain immediately, but it can address the underlying cause of toothache within a few days of repeated use. Before brushing your teeth and with an empty stomach, take one Tbsp of oil into your mouth and swish it around for 10-20 minutes until the oil has turned milky white. Then spit out. Most any food oil can do, but sesame and sunflower oils are traditional and the most popular.

Tooth Abscess

When a tooth gets infected, pus can form in the tissues between the jawbone and the tooth. It can result in pain that is dull to excruciating. A bacterial infection is usually the cause, with the bacteria gaining entry from tooth decay, periodontal disease, or other damage to the teeth. Warning! A tooth infection or abscess can quickly spread to the rest of the body and can even be fatal. Consult a dentist early on or if the infection worsens.

BEST REMEDIES:

- **Garlic:** For toothache or a developing abscess, take a clove of garlic, place it on the affected tooth, and gently bite down on it so that the garlic juices begin to spread over the area. Pain may increase at first but should soon subside entirely. Garlic's sulfur and other components may be able to kill off the infection entirely.
- **Oil Pulling:** The ancient practice of oil pulling is finding renewed fame for its ability to pull toxins out of the body. It may not relieve pain immediately, but it can address the abscess within a few days of repeated use. Before brushing your teeth and with an empty stomach, take one Tbsp of oil into your mouth and swish it around for 10-20 minutes until the oil has turned milky white. Then spit out. Most any food oil can do, but sesame and sunflower oils are traditional and the most popular.
- **Hydrogen Peroxide:** Pour out about a half-tablespoon of 3% hydrogen peroxide and hold it in your mouth for several minutes, gently swishing the solution across the affected tooth to kill off the infection. Repeat twice daily. You can also soak a cotton ball in hydrogen peroxide and hold it against the tooth. Be aware that hydrogen peroxide is a mild bleaching agent.

Tooth Infection

When a tooth gets infected, pus can form in the tissues between the jawbone and the tooth. It can result in pain that is dull to excruciating. A bacterial infection is usually the cause, with the bacteria gaining entry from tooth decay, periodontal disease, or other damage to the teeth. Warning! A tooth infection or abscess can quickly spread to the rest of the body and can even be fatal. Consult a dentist early on or if the infection worsens.

BEST REMEDIES:

- **Garlic:** For toothache or a developing abscess, take a clove of garlic, place it on the affected tooth, and gently bite down on it so that the garlic juices begin to spread over the area. Pain may increase at first but should soon subside entirely. Garlic's sulfur and other components may be able to kill off the infection entirely.

- **Oil Pulling:** The ancient practice of oil pulling is finding renewed fame for its ability to pull toxins out of the body. It may not relieve pain immediately, but it can address the abscess within a few days of repeated use. Before brushing your teeth and with an empty stomach, take one Tbsp of oil into your mouth and swish it around for 10-20 minutes until the oil has turned milky white. Then spit out. Most any food oil can do, but sesame and sunflower oils are traditional and the most popular.
- **Hydrogen Peroxide:** Pour out about a half-tablespoon of 3% hydrogen peroxide and hold it in your mouth for several minutes, gently swishing the solution across the affected tooth to kill off the infection. Repeat twice daily. You can also soak a cotton ball in hydrogen peroxide and hold it against the tooth. Be aware that hydrogen peroxide is a mild bleaching agent.

U

Ulcers

A stomach ulcer or peptic ulcer may form in the stomach or duodenum. An ulcer will likely result in pain, usually around meals, and may be accompanied by nausea, vomiting with blood, loss of appetite, bloating, and other symptoms. Most cases (more than 70%) are caused by the Helicobacter pylori bacteria.

BEST REMEDY:
- **Cayenne:** It may sound a bit crazy, but people have had great success in curing difficult ulcers with cayenne. Cayenne capsules are available, but for a direct approach, drink a teaspoon of powdered cayenne pepper in a glass of hot water once a day.

Urinary Tract Infections

Bacteria in the kidneys, bladder, or urethra can create a urinary tract infection (UTI), which can be painful, especially during urination. The pain and discomfort can be remedied at home, but serious or reoccurring pain should be addressed with a doctor.

BEST REMEDIES:
- **Apple Cider Vinegar:** A day or two of twice daily ACV tonics should halt a bladder infection, but continue for a few days afterward to make sure—take 1-2 tablespoons apple cider vinegar, unsweetened, in a tall glass of water. Also, taking a bath with one cup of ACV added to the warm water can be very healing.
- **Cranberry:** Cranberry pills and unsweetened cranberry juice can put an end to bladder infections.
- **D-Mannose:** D-mannose seems to be the active ingredient in cranberry juice that prevents and may stop a

bladder infection. You can find D-mannose pills at some health food stores and pharmacies.

- **Alka Seltzer:** Take Alka Seltzer as directed to relieve bladder infection symptoms quickly. May not kill off the infection, but the relief is well worth it! Combine with another UTI remedy for a cure.
- **Apple Cider Vinegar and Baking Soda:** Two or three times a day, drink a large glass of water with 1-2 tablespoons of apple cider vinegar and an eighth of a teaspoon of baking soda (watch out for the fizz!).
- **Baking Soda:** Half a teaspoon of baking soda dissolved in a glass of water 2-3 times a day can provide instant relief from the burning. It will eventually remedy a bladder infection by restoring an alkaline balance to your body.
- **Sea Salt:** A one-dose remedy (and no more than once!). Add a teaspoon of sea salt to a large glass of water and drink. Very effective, especially if combined with other UTI remedies.

Vaginal Warts/Genital Warts

The highly contagious HPV virus can cause genital warts in the exposed person. Very small warts or larger clusters can form throughout the genital and anal area, and they can spread HPV to sexual partners through skin-to-skin contact.

BEST REMEDIES:
- **Apple Cider Vinegar:** An exceedingly popular remedy, apple cider vinegar (ACV) can be very effective within a few days. Simply soak a cotton ball in ACV and apply to the warts. You can use a band-aid to hold the cotton to the wart for a few hours at a time. Okay for internal use, though there will be significant discomfort at first.
- **Garlic:** Scrape the skin off one edge of a clove of garlic and apply it directly to the genital wart. It will burn, but you can leave it on the wart for perhaps an hour at a time, reapplying several times throughout the day.

Vaginosis

An imbalance in the body's natural variety and amount of bacteria results in bacterial vaginosis, the most common type of bacterial infection. An unpleasant "fishy" smell and off-white vaginal discharge are the primary symptoms.

BEST REMEDIES:
- **Hydrogen Peroxide:** 3% hydrogen peroxide, usually mixed with equal parts water, can be used as a douche or applied to a tampon (for temporary use, maybe 20-30 minutes).
- **Acidophilus:** Acidophilus pills can be taken orally and inserted vaginally to add healthy bacteria to the vagina and

restore your natural balance. Acidophilus is a normal part of the vaginal environment.

- **Folic Acid:** 800 mcg of folic acid taken orally on a daily basis seems to strengthen the body and restore balance to the vaginal environment so that the smell and discharge go away. The CDC recommends at least 400mcg daily for all women, regardless.
- **Boric Acid:** A capsule of boric acid inserted into the vagina can quickly stop the smell and discharge. Finding boric acid can be tricky, but your pharmacist should be able to order it for you.
- **Probiotics:** Probiotic pills (they should be refrigerated!) are available that specifically target BV and similar conditions. Not all probiotics will have the same effect, so take your time in finding the right probiotic mix.
- **Yogurt:** Plain yogurt with live cultures can be eaten or applied directly (try filling a tampon applicator) to restore your supply of healthy bacteria and stop the odor and discharge.

Viral Conjunctivitis

Conjunctivitis, better known as 'pink eye', is a viral infection that causes irritation, watering, reddening of the eyes, and a distinct pinkness of the eye's conjunctiva (the combined area at the edge of the eye and on the inside of the eyelid). A bacterial form is also possible.

BEST REMEDIES:
- **Apple Cider Vinegar:** Mix about two teaspoons of unpasteurized apple cider vinegar in a cup of water, then dip a cotton pad or soft cloth in it to wash the eyelid inside and out. You can place a few drops of the water mixture in the eye as well. Repeat every few hours until the conjunctivitis is all gone, usually 2-3 days.
- **Green Tea Bags:** Put two green tea bags in a cup of hot water and allow the tea to brew and then cool somewhat, then apply each bag to an eye. Rewarm in the water and

continue for about 10 minutes. Repeat every few hours until healed, usually 2-3 days.

- **Colloidal Silver:** Place a drop of colloidal silver in the affected eye 2-3 times a day until symptoms are gone.
- **Sea Salt:** Combine a tablespoon of sea salt in a cup of water and apply 2-3 drops to the corners of your eyes first thing in the morning and last thing at night.
- **Black Tea Bag:** Make a cup of black tea and allow it to cool a bit. Then apply the tea bag to the eye and keep it there for ten minutes or so. Repeat every few hours for the 1-3 days it will take to clear up the conjunctivitis.

Virus - Flu

Influenza, the common flu, is an annual threat to worldwide health, especially among the youngest and oldest among us. Accompanied by fever and aching as well as the typical cold symptoms, the flu can progress to become pneumonia, a far more serious condition.

BEST REMEDIES:
- **Apple Cider Vinegar:** Take a tablespoon each of apple cider vinegar and honey in a warm but not hot glass of water up to three times a day to relieve all flu symptoms, including sore throat.
- **Hydrogen Peroxide:** At the first sign of the flu, lie on your side and put a few drops of 3% hydrogen peroxide in your ear, and then let it sit for several minutes. Then empty out that ear and repeat on the other side. Hydrogen peroxide's antiviral properties seem to cut the flu virus down before it can take hold.
- **Grapefruit Seed Extract:** A few drops of grapefruit seed extract, taken as directed, can stop a flu in its tracks and greatly reduce flu symptoms.
- **Hydrogen Peroxide Inhalation:** While it should be undertaken carefully, using an emptied nasal spray bottle to inhale 3% hydrogen peroxide can open up airways and reduce flu symptoms. (Be sure to first sterilize the spray

bottle with boiling water.) Point the spray bottle in your mouth and at the back of your throat, and while inhaling sharply pump 4-6 sprays of the hydrogen peroxide. Repeat 4-6 times a day.

Vomiting, Severe

Can't stop throwing up? We have one very fast-working Ayurvedic remedy involving onions and peppermint tea, with a couple of other remedies thrown in for good measure!

BEST REMEDIES:
- **Black Tea:** Brew a cup of black tea using two tea bags to create an extra strong cup of tea (add a teaspoon of honey, if you like). Within a few minutes of sipping the tea, your nausea should vanish.
- **Honey:** Eating a teaspoon of honey can stop nausea and vomiting in no time at all. Feel free to also add a bit of honey to food as you first begin to eat again. It will help the foods go down.
- **Onion Juice:** Prepare peppermint tea and allow to cool while you grate an onion. Squeeze the pulp through cheesecloth to make 1 tablespoon of Fresh Onion Juice. Hold your nose and swallow the onion juice, then follow with just 1 tablespoon of peppermint tea. Wait ten minutes. Take another tablespoon of peppermint tea. Wait 15 minutes. This remedy should stop vomiting within 15 minutes. The peppermint tea also helps to re-hydrate you.

Warts

The HPV virus can cause the cauliflower-like bumps on the skin that we call warts. Mostly found on the hands and feet, warts can be contagious and can return even after they have vanished.

BEST REMEDIES:

- **Banana Peel:** Far and away the most popular wart remedy, this one is also one of the easiest. Simply rub the inside of a little piece of a banana peel on a wart every night. You should see results within one to two weeks. The banana peel's ample potassium supply kills off the wart bit by bit, with no pain!
- **Apple Cider Vinegar:** Apple Cider Vinegar (ACV) is also a very popular wart remedy. Soak a bit of cotton in ACV, apply it to the wart, and secure it with a band-aid. You can replace the cotton with a new soak once or twice a day. In a couple of weeks, your wart should be gone.
- **Voodoo:** There are a few variations on "Voodoo" remedies to cure warts, but the most popular seems to be this one. Take a raw potato and cut out a slice, rub that slice all over the wart, and then bury the slice somewhere—telling no one where you've buried it! In a couple of weeks, with no more treatments, your wart will be gone.
- **Duct Tape:** The duct tape remedy for warts gets a lot of support all across the internet. The idea is simply to cover the wart with a strip of duct tape, choking the wart's oxygen supply. Whenever the tape gets loose, gently scrape at the top of the wart and then put a new piece of tape on.
- **Hydrogen Peroxide:** Dab a cotton swab in 3% hydrogen peroxide and apply it to the wart for a few minutes. Be ready for some discomfort. Repeat daily or a couple of

times a day until the wart dies off, often within several days.

- **Tea Tree Oil:** Apply a drop of tea tree oil to a wart and then cover it with a band-aid. Re-apply once or twice a day. Within about two weeks, the wart should fall right off.
- **Vitamin E:** Vitamin E liquid supplements can be used internally and externally to treat a wart. Take the pills as directed. Additionally, once a day puncture one of the pills and apply the Vitamin E oil directly to the wart, then cover with a bandage.
- **Banana Peel and Duct Tape:** Combining two of our most popular wart remedies into one might be the best bet. Rub the inside of a little piece of a banana peel on a wart and keep it in place with a strip of duct tape applied so as to completely cover the wart. Whenever the tape gets loose, throw it away, gently scrape at the top of the wart, and then put new pieces of banana peel and tape on.

Weight Loss Remedies

We are all looking for a simpler or more effective weigh to lose weight, whether our weight loss goals are large or small. Fewer calories and more activity is the way to go, for sure, but some natural way to boost metabolism, reduce cravings, increase energy levels, and improve our nutrition would go a long way in helping us to reach our weight loss goals!

BEST REMEDIES:
- **Apple Cider Vinegar:** Even when taking apple cider vinegar (ACV) for entirely different reasons, people often report losing weight with no other change than adding ACV to their diets. Two options: First option, mix 2 teaspoons of ACV in 16 ounces of water that you'll sip throughout the day. You will be keeping your pH in an alkalized state by sipping this highly diluted dosage. Usually 1-2 tall glasses of the concoction are all you'll need

each day. Second option, take the ACV tonic three times a day with meals—one teaspoon of ACV in a large glass of water. Increase the amount of ACV to 1-2 tablespoons per glass as your body tolerates it.

- **Coconut Oil:** Adding up to a tablespoonful of cold pressed coconut oil to your daily diet can help to reduce cravings. Otherwise, its effectiveness as a diet aid is something of a mystery, but reports are very favorable!
- **Master Cleanses:** That old water-cooler favorite, the Master Cleanse, has been a successful means for many people to lose weight quickly and restore the body's overall health so as to keep the weight off. Find a dependable online source for the Cleanse's rigid procedure.
- **Honey and Cinnamon:** Add a combination of honey and tea to your daily diet to reduce cravings and lose weight. Try a teaspoon of honey and a couple good shakes of cinnamon in a mug of warm water for a breakfast tea. Or add the same to a slice of toast. A great, energetic way to start the day!

X-Z

Yeast Infections

A vaginal yeast infection is characterized by burning, itching, soreness, pain during intercourse and/or urination, and vaginal discharge that looks rather like cottage cheese. A diagnosis is confirmed through identification of the yeast under a microscope from a specimen scraped from the vaginal area.

BEST REMEDIES:

- **Apple Cider Vinegar:** Apple Cider Vinegar (ACV) may burn a touch at first, but then it brings lasting relief. Wet a cotton pad, cloth, or cotton ball in an equal parts mixture of water and ACV. Apply it to the labia or any external skin where itching and irritation are occurring, and hold it in place for a few minutes. Generally, Earth Clinic doesn't recommend douching, but many have found relief from internal symptoms by filling a douche with 2-3 tablespoons of apple cider vinegar and warm water, or you can also soak a tampon in ACV for internal use as well.

- **Yogurt:** Simple eating unflavored yogurt can end a yeast infection. Look for a brand with active cultures and free of artificial sweeteners. You can also use an applicator to apply the yogurt directly to your vagina for instant, soothing relief.

- **Boric Acid:** Boric acid suppositories can be used to restore your body's natural balance. You most likely will have to fill your own caplets, but you can easily get these and boric acid powder from the pharmacy. Insert a 600mg suppository each night, usually for about two weeks, for a lasting remedy. (NOT FOR INGESTION!)

- **Garlic:** Use a needle to run a string through a clove of garlic, and insert the garlic into your vagina with the string trailing. Great for overnight use.

- **Hydrogen Peroxide:** Wet a cotton pad, cloth, or cotton ball in an equal parts mixture of water and 3% hydrogen peroxide. Apply it to the labia or any external skin where itching and irritation are occurring, and hold it in place for a few minutes. Generally, Earth Clinic doesn't recommend douching, but many have found relief from internal symptoms by filling a douche with 1 tablespoon of hydrogen peroxide and warm water, or you can also soak a tampon in an equal parts mix of water and hydrogen peroxide for internal use as well.
- **Acidophilus:** Acidophilus is a bacteria that naturally occurs in the human body, including in the vagina. To reduce yeast levels and restore your body's natural balance, you can take acidophilus capsules available at the pharmacy. Use as directed for a long-term yeast infection cure. For fast relief, some women will insert a tablet vaginally in addition to the oral route.
- **Apple Cider Vinegar and Salt:** Try taking a warm bath to soothe and cleanse externally and internally. Add a half-cup of apple cider vinegar and a cup of sea salt or other salt to the bathwater.

APPENDICES

Appendix 1:
General and Specific Notes of Caution

Of course, you have already seen our obligatory legal proviso on the first pages, cautioning you that no matter how carefully we have put this book together, you should always check with a doctor who understands your complete medical history. As much as the folks behind Earth Clinic love and rely on natural remedies in our own lives, we definitely encourage you to consult with a local medical expert for any reasonably serious condition. At the least, they can give you a more definite diagnosis and additional knowledge about the standard medical understanding of your condition.

However, there are some specific concerns you should keep in mind as well, whenever you are using natural remedies.

Side Effects
Any change in your diet or routine can have side effects. Even the very natural remedies we advocate can trigger allergies or unexpected reactions. So do please be careful, and note both the positive and negative effects any home remedy seems to have on your specific condition and overall health.

Hydrogen Peroxide
A number of our remedies feature hydrogen peroxide in one of two forms—standard 3% hydrogen peroxide as you'll find on the typical store shelf, and 35% hydrogen peroxide, so called Food Grade Hydrogen Peroxide.

CAUTION: Food grade, or 35% hydrogen peroxide is very dangerous and absolutely must be diluted before use!

If not otherwise noted, whenever we speak of hydrogen peroxide we mean of the 3% variety. If you choose to use the more concentrated 35% version, be certain to understand the necessary dilution procedures and be very careful in its usage.

You Are Unique!

You already knew that about yourself, we know! Who doesn't like to hear how special they are, even if it's only in our mother's eyes? In this case, however, it is definitely true. As we said above about seeing your own doctor, we say again in regards to the Earth Clinic Community. It's full of tremendous advice, but as much as we'd like to, not a one of us knows you or your specific health needs. That's what Earth Clinic is about, though, empowering each of us to take control of our own health to figure out exactly what it is that ails us, and what it is that our own body needs to get over that ailment and back on the path to better health!

In that light, please remember that different remedies will work for different people; so please don't be discouraged if the first remedy on the list has no obvious effect on your condition. It is often worthwhile to try several of the top remedies to find the one that works best for your particular condition and overall biology (sometimes, even if the first one works pretty well). Doctors do the same for chronic conditions, looking for the drug that works best for you, with the fewest side effects. It's just that our "drugs" have far fewer side effects to begin with!

Appendix 2:
Apple Cider Vinegar

As our oldest and most popular remedy, apple cider vinegar deserves its own moment in the spotlight.

The Apple Cider Vinegar Tonic
Over the course of this book's many remedies, apple cider vinegar and especially the ACV Tonic come up time and again. There's a good reason that this site got its very organic start with apple cider vinegar (ACV)—it serves time and again to repair and restore the body after all kinds of damage and illnesses.

However, not every person's condition is the same, and naturally then neither is the exact same tonic right for every person. If you've scanned through quite a lot of the remedies in this book, you'll notice that the ACV Tonic is often described differently from one condition to the next. We have done so on purpose.

For certain, the basic ACV Tonic is always the same, but how it is diluted, what it is mixed with, and when it is taken can be an important variable in getting the best health benefits from this natural remedy. Some conditions are exacerbated by sugars, so we advise against sweetening the tonic; whereas at other times a teaspoon of honey will provide a perfect complement to the treatment, adding its own inherent health benefits to the mix. A digestive condition is going to often demand that the tonic be consumed alongside meals, while a more pervasive or whole health condition might be best served by a more diluted form of the tonic taken throughout the day to alkalize and smooth out the body's cycles.

In any case, let us here and now present the basic ACV Tonic recipes for general consultation:

ORIGINAL ACV TONIC
1 tsp and up to 2 tbsp unpasteurized apple cider vinegar
1 large glass of water (8-12 oz.)
1 tsp natural sweetener (optional)

This version of the tonic is mixed and ordinarily taken just before or along with meals, 1-3 times a day. When it comes to natural sweeteners, honey is probably ideal since it offers substantial health benefits of its own. Natural maple syrup likewise has many proponents, whereas refined sugar also offers sweetness but little if any other health benefit. Any natural sweetener, however, will do just fine. Alternatively, some prefer to forgo a separate sweetener and simply mix their ACV in with apple juice, apple cider, or another drink that blends well with the cider vinegar. The possibilities are endless, the point is just to get the stuff into your system and your dietary habits.

MODERN ACV TONIC
2 tsp unpasteurized apple cider vinegar
16 ounces water

Mix together in a container and refrigerate, pouring yourself a glassful whenever you are thirsty. Ordinarily a couple of glasses a day will take care of your general health needs. This version is ideal for those who are particularly concerned about maintaining an alkalizing diet for overall health.

ACV TONIC WITH BAKING SODA
1/8 tsp baking soda (sodium bicarbonate)
1-6 tsp apple cider vinegar
8-16 oz water

Add an eighth of a teaspoon of baking soda to either of the standard ACV tonics found above. Be careful! When you initially combine the vinegar and baking soda, a natural reaction will cause it to fizz up somewhat dramatically. Once the reaction settles, you can drink this version of the tonic as above for an additional alkalizing boost.

What Sort of ACV?

In this book, we have glossed over the extended discussion concerning what to look for in a good apple cider vinegar, in the interest of brevity. Now that we have a little space, let's take the topic for a short walk.

In some cases, white vinegar will do just as well as any apple cider vinegar. However, whenever you ingest the remedy, apple cider vinegar has vastly superior benefits over just about any other form of vinegar, according to our community reports. Best of all is unpasteurized apple cider vinegar. Many such brands exist, though they are hard to find at most grocery stores. Just be sure to get genuine apple cider vinegar, naturally fermented. Distilled vinegar with apple flavoring is a very cheap but common substitute.

Pasteurization of ACV, just as with milk and other products, means that it is heated to kill off any potential pathogens—whether they are there or not. Fortunately, ACV has strong antibiotic properties, so this step is unnecessary. Beyond being unneeded, this heating also destroys or alters a number of valuable components of natural apple cider vinegar. For this reason, we strongly encourage the extra bit of effort it takes to find unpasteurized apple cider vinegar. Years of experience and thousands of reports on Earth Clinic have illustrated real merit in making this distinction.

Organic versions of apple cider vinegar are also available and likewise admirable, probably protecting your health if not directly providing it any additional benefit. All in all though, unpasteurized is the simple gold standard when it comes to apple cider vinegar.

ABOUT THE EDITOR

Daniel P. Kray has worked for several years on the Earth Clinic website after being hand-selected by the site's founder as someone whose vital energy exactly matched that of the Earth Clinic community. The collaboration was a natural choice and has continued through several productive years and ventures. That includes helping to launch the Body Axis publishing venture to share the ever-growing harvest of Earth Clinic knowledge with an even wider community.

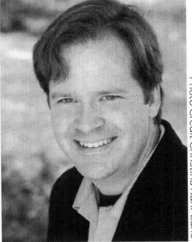

Along with other publishing credits, Dan has been senior writer and editor for a number of leading internet sites. A graduate of Williams College, his experience in publishing, education, travel (six continents), and knowledge of biology, medicine, and exercise theory prepared him for the continuing Body Axis project. He is a resident of a bucolic New York village.

Photo Credit Christina Rahr Lane

Made in the USA
San Bernardino, CA
27 July 2015